Praise

"Aanna is a dedicated follower of Jesus whose love for Him pours out passionately on these pages. She addresses important topics in an accessible, shame-free way and draws her darling readers closer to God."–Lori Wilhite, author of *Leading and Loving It: Encouragement for Pastors' Wives and Women in Leadership*

"*Darling* opens up a much needed conversation for Christian women in our culture today. Aanna's straight forward approach shares a beautiful platform of education to avert potential sexual disillusionment and disappointment. Working in a sexual health clinic, I see firsthand the havoc that closed communication about sexuality can bring. The wonder of sex can be privately explored through the pages of *Darling*, setting the stage for God's design of intimacy between a husband and wife."–Karolyn Schrage RN, BSN, Executive Director of Life Choices, Joplin, MO

"From mothers of daughters, to couples in premarital counseling, to single women, any woman will be educated, blessed, and empowered by the words in these pages. Aanna Greer has done a great job of painting a picture of godly sexuality."–Jason Epperson, Senior Pastor of CU Christian Church

"Sex–it's a three-letter word that gets a lot of attention. Unfortunately, for most Christian women, much of that attention can be summarized by the earliest messages we hear, 'Don't do it...Don't give away your virginity...Just wait.' There are, of course, good reasons for part of that message, but where is the message that rejoices in sexual intimacy? 'Yes, be sexual in your marriage...Delight in the body God gave you...Enjoy the wonder of sex!' Aanna has courageously and wisely supplied what has been missing."–Julie Gariss, Co-Director of the Life and Ministry Preparation Center, Ozark Christian College

Darling

DARLING

A Woman's Guide to Godly Sexuality

Aanna Greer

HATCHBOOK

Darling: A Woman's Guide to Godly Sexuality
By Aanna Greer
Published by Hatchbook Publishing
Joplin, MO, 64801
© 2017 Aanna Greer

Cover design by Sarah Hester.

ISBN 978-0-9990545-0-5

For Logan

dar·ling

'därliNG/

noun

    used as an affectionate form of address to a beloved person.

    a dearly loved person.

adjective

    beloved.

    dearly loved.

    very pleasing or attractive.

Define yourself radically as one beloved by God. This is the true self. Every other identity is illusion.

                                 —*Brennan Manning*

Contents

Preface

One crisp fall evening my husband and I went for a walk in the country, and I was spitting mad.

Over the course of a few weeks I had heard several women's stories that were both alarming and upsetting. It seemed that in an effort to keep women innocent, women are also often kept ignorant of the details of anatomy, sexuality, and sex. And even though nearly everyone is exposed to sexual content in the media, there is very little accurate and healthy information given at the same time.

My husband turned to me and said simply, "Why don't you do something about it?"

With over ten years of youth and college ministry experience, a stint teaching sex education in the public school system, and a penchant for obsessively reading on the subject, I decided to tackle the issue. What I discovered was an enormous collection of good and helpful information out there for people who wanted it. My goal became connecting women to that information so that they would be knowledgeable and feel empowered about issues of womanhood and sexuality.

As the oldest of seven sisters, I know firsthand the kind of helpful tips and easy advice that can be found in the company of other women. Because of this, I also interviewed a group of brave women who wanted to be able to offer you this kind of sisterly conversation about sexuality. Their names have been changed for the sake of anonymity so that they could share their stories uncut and raw. Along with these helpful sources, I will share the advice of Dr. Cheryl Fogarty, OB/GYN, whose practical medical advice is eye-opening and easy to understand.

The first part of this book is about godly sexuality and what it means to be healthy and whole as a sexual, single, and chaste woman. The second part of the book is for those of you who see marriage on the horizon and need to start preparing your heart, mind, and body for sex. The third part of this book is for married women, with helpful tips for navigating the joy and the euphoria, the problems and the pain that you may encounter in your sex life.

All along the way, I kept thinking about the fact that God was the one who made our bodies, created sex, and invented sexuality. I wondered, "What does God think about sex?" The answer to that question seemed to me to be the solution to all our questions and troubles concerning sexuality. But in the end, I realized that the better question is, "What does sex tell us about God?" And the answer is astonishing. My hope and prayer is that in the pages of this book and through the experience of participating in your sexuality in the intended, complete, and most pleasurable way, you will get a more intimate and revealing glimpse of God himself.

Much love,
Aanna Greer

Introduction

This book is not about being a virgin.

In recent history, Christians have obsessed over the idea of virginity. From abstinence programs to purity ring rituals to sermons and devotional books about sex, Christian leaders emphasize virginity as the primary way to please God with your sexuality. The idea is that if you make it to marriage without having sex, then you will please God, enjoy a superior sex life in marriage, and escape a myriad of evils, from STDs to a broken heart.

You're either a virgin or you're not. Pure or impure. In or out.

This idea has failed us in numerous ways. Christian women sometimes conclude that sex must be bad, that it corrupts purity, or that it is to be feared. Christian virgins who enter marriage suddenly deal with crushing guilt because of their regular sexual activity. Women who have once had sex outside marriage view themselves as outsiders of the Christian life, purity as out of reach as their lost virginity.

But sex was created by God. He envisioned and crafted it—much like an artist would imagine and execute a painting—then gave it to every man and woman. Within this gift, humanity would discover gender, romance, marriage, and sex—four components that interlock to form the essence of sexuality. It exists within the nature of every woman, like her heart or her soul; she doesn't have to be having sex to be a sexual being. God gives every woman the ability to feel and respond sexually, to have sex, to conceive and bear children, and to act upon her sexuality in a way that pleases God.

God wants you to partake in his good gift in a way that maximizes your experience of it. For centuries, Christians have called this being chaste—engaging your sexuality in the way that God intended when he first created it. We can be chaste whether we're single and patiently abstaining from sex, engaged and eagerly preparing for it, or married and joyfully partaking in it.

We do this both because of who God is and because of who we are. In a startling scene from the book of Exodus, God reveals his physical form to Moses and gives humanity a description of his own character: "The Lord, the Lord, a God merciful and gracious, slow to anger, and abounding in *steadfast love* and faithfulness" (Ex. 34:6 ESV, emphasis added). God has loved us with an everlasting love. In fact, whenever Scripture uses the word "godly," it refers not to those who are blameless or good, but to those who have "genuinely laid hold of God's steadfast love."[1] Because of God's perfect love displayed to us through Jesus' death on the cross, our lives are no longer defined by being pure or impure, in or out, virgin or not a virgin. Our lives are defined by the love of God for us.

Merriam-Webster defines "darling" as "a dearly loved person; greatly loved; very pleasing."[2] A darling is someone who knows who she is, who is beloved by a good Creator, and who bravely lives life in accordance with that reality. Her identity is no longer defined by the good or bad things she's done; it's not defined by her sexuality or her singleness, her accomplishments or failures, or her ability to have a boyfriend or a child. A darling is one who has laid hold of God's steadfast love.

This book is about being a darling.

Part One

Single Darlings

1

God's Design for Sex

God wanted to reveal Himself and the value He places on intimate loving relationships, so He created sexuality.
—Dr. Douglas E. Rosenau

Recognize the true goodness of God's creation; things as they were in the Garden of Eden are things at their most nourishing, they are things as they are meant to be.
—Lauren F. Winner

There is a simple way to discover God's design for sex.

We can learn everything we need to know about the best kind of sex and love and romance and intimacy from taking a look at how things were in the Garden of Eden.

The idea is that when we want to know God's will about something, we can look at how he first created things, at the perfect world before sin entered it, to see what he ultimately had in mind. And in fact, whenever Jesus was asked about marriage and sex, he pointed back to the Garden of Eden. The apostle Paul did the same thing many times. So we go back to the very beginning, when God first created a man and a woman and put them together, to find out what he thinks about sexuality.

The Design of Sex

Let's take a look at the creation account in the first and second chapter of Genesis:

> Then God said, "Let us make human beings in our image, to be like us. They will reign over the fish in the sea, the birds in the sky, the livestock, all the wild animals on the earth, and the small animals that scurry along the ground."
>
> So God created human beings in his own image.
> In the image of God he created them;
> male and female he created them.
> —Genesis 1:26–27 NLT
>
> Then the Lord God said, "It is not good for the man to be alone. I will make a helper who is just right for him."
> —Genesis 2:18 NLT
>
> So the Lord God caused the man to fall into a deep sleep. While the man slept, the Lord God took out one of the man's ribs and closed up the opening. Then the Lord God made a woman from the rib, and he brought her to the man.
>
> "At last!" the man exclaimed. "This one is bone from my bone, and flesh from my flesh! She will be called 'woman,' because she was taken from 'man.'"
>
> This explains why a man leaves his father and mother and is joined to his wife, and the two are united into one.
> —Genesis 2:21-24 NLT
>
> Then God looked over all he had made, and he saw that it was very good!
> —Genesis 1:31 NLT

This is it! This is what God thinks about sex, what he made it for, how he wanted it to be used. This tells us what we need to know about sex and becomes a solid foundation for answering any questions we come across.

Sex Is Good

"God saw everything that he had made, and behold, it was very good" (Gen. 1:31 ESV). Because we find sex in God's original plan for the earth, the first thing we can observe is that sex is good! Sex is not an accident or a perversion of God's creation, but something that he created on purpose and then joyfully gave to humanity. Sex is good and is a part of God's plan for men and women.

Sex Is For Marriage

The second thing we find is that sex is for marriage. The very first verse about marriage explains that "a man leaves his father and mother and is joined to his wife, and the two are united into one" (Gen. 2:24 NLT). After a woman and a man have decided to pledge themselves to one another in love and service forever, sex—being "united into one"—is a gift from God to be used to sweeten and solidify this bond.

The last sentence of Fitzgerald's exquisite novel *The Great Gatsby* is, "And so we beat on, boats against the current, borne back ceaselessly into the past."[3] If you were to read that sentence, without having read the book, would you understand the breadth of the beauty, meaning, and richness of the entire story? Of course not! But having sex outside marriage is like reading the last line of a book and thinking you understand the whole of it. When God created sex, he created it within the context of unconditional love and a promise of faithfulness. Sex loses its meaning when you take it out of marriage.

Sex Is for Two People

The third thing we find is that sex is for two people. God made community part of the essence of sex. In the act of sexual intercourse, two people come together, for "it is not good for the man to be alone" (Gen. 2:18 NIV). But while sex does not include fewer than two people, it also does not include more, and this concept becomes a good plumb line for discerning healthy sexual practices.

If sexual interaction ever includes more than two people (an affair, threesomes, pornography, orgies), then it is no longer within the boundaries of proper use. Although sex should never include more than two people, it also shouldn't include less (masturbation; being disengaged during the sexual act). Sex was made for two people in marriage, and both are to fully engage and participate in the act in order to experience sex the way God intended.

Sex Is for a Man and a Woman

The last thing we find is that sex is between a man and a woman. "In the image of God he created them; male and female he created them" (Gen. 1:27 NLT). In this perfect example of sex, it occurs between a man and a woman. This is the basis for the Christian theology concerning homosexuality, but it is part of a much larger issue.

When God created sexuality, he made it to be experienced between a man and a woman. What this tells us is that God created gender and that it's an incredibly significant aspect of humanity. Genesis 1:27 is saying that through gender God most fully displays his own image. He can't be fully understood in man, he can't be fully seen in woman, but together we have a more complete picture of what God is like. That means that embracing our gender is a vital part of embracing our sexuality and God's purpose for it in our lives.

The Purpose of Marriage

Sex may be God's way of calling us to connect with each other.
—Gary Thomas

Remember, God imagined and crafted sex the way an artist would imagine and then execute a painting. He designed sex to be good, to be for marriage, to be for two people, and to be between a man and a woman. But why did he do it? What was the purpose of sex?

Just as God used great care in designing sex, he also had great purpose in creating it. There are four distinct reasons why God created sex, with a fifth that overshadows and clarifies all the rest.

Marriage

Just as sex is designed for marriage, it also finds its purpose in marriage. One purpose is that it's the best (and probably only) place for sex to thrive. As Tim Keller says, "According to the Bible, a covenant is necessary for sex. It creates a place of security for vulnerability and intimacy."[4] Anyone who has had much experience or done much study on the subject knows that vulnerability and intimacy make up the bedrock of a good sex life. Without it, sex will never be more than a few moments of fun. Marriage helps you enjoy better sex.

The second way that sex finds its purpose in marriage is by providing a way to renew the marriage vows on a regular basis. It's a reminder to couples of their promises and sacred bond, and gives them a way to celebrate and honor it often. Sex helps couples enjoy a better marriage.

Unity

When a couple has sex, literally making it difficult to tell where one person ends and the other begins, we find a truth that permeates the physical, mental, spiritual, and emotional.[5] With every orgasm that a man and wife experience together, their brains receive a shot of dopamine, a naturally occurring chemical that builds and strengthens bonds created between two people. As the years go by, the very act of sex will be the tool that fuses your brain to your spouse, physically and mentally tying you to each other. When you have sex, God declares that you are one spiritually and that no one should try to separate you, not even yourselves (Matthew 19:6). Even a couple who has a one-night stand feels an emotional connection that is hard to break, though there is nothing holding them together in a legal, relational, or social way. God desires sexual practices that create real and lasting unity, one of the most fulfilling experiences in human existence.

Procreation

Sex was intended by God for procreation. An important aspect of relaying a true picture of the love of God is to communicate its creative nature. Whenever and wherever God loves, something beautiful and new will come into existence. And while sex doesn't always have to lead to procreation, it can't be denied that God's vision for sex includes the possibility of procreation. Love should beget love. It should overflow until it spreads, blessing the community.

Pleasure

God wanted sex to be pleasurable. Without pleasure, there would be an insinuation that we may have a relationship with God but not necessarily enjoy it. However, the truth is that with God "to know him is to love him."[6] Once we understand this, "sexual pleasure in the service of God is doxological."[7] Godly sex will embrace pleasure, for both husband and wife, as a means of glorifying God. It's a way to declare that endless pleasure can be found in God's presence (see Ps. 16:11). He is to be desired.

God's Plan Revealed

When a man unites with his wife in holiness, the Shekinah
[glory of God] is between them in the mystery of man and
woman.
　　　　　　　–Nahmanides

It's not hard for any person to discover the purposes of sex–pleasure, bonding, a seal of love, the creation of a child. Over the centuries, these are the things that men and women have consistently found in sex. But two thousand years ago something–someone–came on the scene to drastically alter the way we understand sex. Our understanding shifted when Jesus made himself human, walked among us and gave his life for us so that we might be forgiven and he could enter our hearts and dwell with us for all eternity.

Therefore a man shall leave his father and mother and hold fast
to his wife, and the two shall become one flesh. This mystery is
profound, and I am saying that it refers to Christ and the
church.
　　　　　　　–Ephesians 5:31-32 ESV

In Ephesians, Paul says that sex was a mystery, but the word "mystery" had a different meaning than the one we use today. Paul uses the word to mean that sex was a mystery *that has now been revealed*. Something kept secret has now been shouted from the rooftops. Like the sun streaming through a skylight into a darkened bedroom, we now see sex more clearly. We see what God really, really had in mind.

God created sex to be a picture of Jesus and the church. When sex is used the way God designed it to be, it's a picture of covenant faithfulness, unconditional love, sacrificial service, and unbridled joy. It's a picture of the gospel.

Each time a woman has sex with her husband–even though he has sinned against her, even though his body is imperfect, even if his personality has been distorted by a tragic childhood or family baggage—she demonstrates the acceptance of God himself.

Each time a husband finds more pleasure in bringing his wife to orgasm than experiencing his own, his action mirrors Christ who loved the church and gave himself up for her.

Each time a man and woman look into each other's eyes and, without saying a word, know in their hearts the complete love they have for each other, they get a glimpse of the kind of love that God has for his Son, the Son for the Spirit, and the Spirit for the Father.

Each time we experience joy through sex (whether by orgasm, the embrace of our best friend, the acceptance of our true selves, or one of life's great joys—the creation of a child), then in that moment we get a taste of what it is to experience the presence of Jesus.

In the act of sex, an act that God knew would be stolen, perverted, abused, overused, and demonized, God distributed among all of us the story of his love—something that we could feel, hear, taste, smell, and see, something to ping our brains when we hear of the cross, the perfect act of love. All so he could dwell with us and we could enjoy his glory forever. That, I think, is the real reason why God created sex.

2

Understanding Your Body

I am pleased by them,
And am not ashamed by them.
For my workmanship are they,
And the strength of my thoughts.
                    —"The Odes of Solomon"

When I was younger, the way I ate, looked, and felt about
myself was largely negative or geared toward making someone
else think I was worthy of love. At some point, the notion of
being made in God's image and for a purpose clicked. Our
bodies are incredible! He made us with such amazing detail, so
purposefully thought out and without mistakes.
                    —Olivia

An amazing and important aspect of your sexuality is your gender. God created all humans to be either male or female, which gives us a rich and complementary spectrum of relationships in this world. Even though each woman is unique, understanding and embracing the idea that you are the type of human that is a woman is a vital part of having a godly sexuality. In this chapter, we'll examine the anatomy of the female reproductive system, ways that you can care for your body, and the basics of male sexual anatomy.

Female Anatomy

Know thyself.

—Ancient Greek proverb

When we were children, our mothers would sit us on their knees and teach us our anatomy. "Can you point to your ears?" "Where's your tongue?" "Wiggle your toes!" But I guess it's too difficult or awkward to teach all of the body parts to children. "Can you point to your vulva?" "Where's your clitoris?" "Can you say vagina?"

But our bodies are "fearfully and wonderfully made," filled with the evidence of God's genius (Ps. 139:14 ESV). It can be a deeply spiritual and significant experience to shed some of our embarrassment about our sexual body parts for the sake of understanding the bodies that God gave us. And while our sexual organs are private and meant to be handled with modesty, that doesn't mean that we can't know and understand them, does it?

I recommend becoming familiar with the names and appearance of all your sexual organs. However, for the sake of simplicity, I'd like to focus on the ones that are most important for understanding yourself and your sexuality:

That tulip-shaped area between your legs is your vulva. (People often refer to this as your vagina, but that's not accurate.) It's naturally covered with dark hair (called pubic hair) and the skin in this area feels soft and puffy.

You'll notice that your vulva is separated down the middle by two "lips." These are your labia majora, and if you peel these back you'll find a second set, your labia minora. These protect the three holes between your legs.

The first hole (the one closest to your front) is your urethra. It's tiny —a little slit—and it's so close to the vagina that many people get the two confused. Your urine comes out of this hole.

The second hole is the opening into your vagina. This is where your blood flows out during your period. Your vagina is about four to six inches long, and it's essentially a tube that runs from the opening up to your uterus. The third hole is your anus, where your bowel movement comes out.

The clitoris is another important part of your body. In normal circumstances, it's tiny, smaller than the tip of your finger, and you can find it by unfolding the lips of your outer and inner labia. You can see where all the folds connect near the top of your vulva. If you think of your vulva as an upside-down tulip, with the lips of your labia as the flower petals, think of your clitoris as the point where all the petals come together at the stem.

Every woman's clitoris is different, but you may be able to see it if you uncover it from all the "petals" and the tiny "hood" that covers it. Again, it will look like the tip of your finger, barely visible.

The clitoris is a shaft, having much the shape of a male penis, that runs almost parallel to your vagina. The part that is visible, which is also the most sensitive part, is considered the head of the shaft. (I think it looks a lot like the tip of a man's penis, although smaller and more delicate.)

The clitoris is an incredibly significant body part, because it's the only organ in the human body whose only purpose is sexual pleasure. Only women have them. God made a small, sensitive piece of your body whose only purpose is to give you sexual pleasure. What does that say about our God? What does that say about the way he wants women to participate in sex? Isn't it lovely and wonderful?

The hymen is a flap of tissue partially covering the entrance to the vagina. Every woman's hymen looks different, but an easy way to describe it is to take your fingers and form an "O" with your thumb and forefinger. Now, using your other hand, pinch the flap of skin connecting your thumb and forefinger. This flap of skin in your "O" is similar to the way your hymen looks in your vagina. There's no known reason for the hymen, although there is much speculation. The important thing to know is that you have one.

The last thing I'll mention is your cervix. So you have your vagina, and at the opening to the vagina is the hymen. Well, at the inner end of your vagina is the opening to your uterus, and this opening is called the cervix. The best way to think of your cervix is like an upside-down turtleneck, with the uterus being the sweater. The cervix's neck can be short and thick and open or long and thin and closed or any variation in between, and it often changes depending on the day. Your cervix protects your uterus from anything unwanted getting inside and also produces a fluid during the times of the month that you are fertile.

So there you have it! The most important parts of your sexual anatomy: vulva, labia majora and minora, vagina, clitoris, hymen, and cervix. All the other parts are important too, but more like supporting cast instead of the main characters.

What's the Big Deal about the Hymen?

The hymen is a subject of confusion and "myth" for a lot of people.

–Elizabeth Lee, MD

Throughout history, people have always linked a woman's hymen with her virginity. Here's the assumption: a hymen completely covers the opening of a woman's vagina until a penis breaks it open during her first experience of sexual intercourse. When a hymen breaks, it will bleed. (In Deuteronomy 22:13–21, there is a law that mentions "proof of a woman's virginity" being the bloody cloth on which a newlywed couple first has sex.) Sometimes, the hymen is crudely referred to as a woman's "cherry," and when a man has sex with her, breaking her hymen, it's referred to as "popping her cherry." Obviously, this sounds kind of awful and violent, but it doesn't have to be like this.

It's strange that this idea still persists because in reality every woman's hymen is different. For some women, the hymen is the shape of a crescent, covering only a small part of the opening. For others, it covers the entire opening except for a small slit. It can be thick or thin, big or small.

Another important fact is that you don't have to have sex to stretch or tear your hymen. It can happen with simple things like tampon usage, gymnastics, or horseback riding.

Obviously, if your hymen only covers part of your vagina, it would be easy for your husband's penis to enter your vagina and would not cause any discomfort or bleeding, even if you are a virgin. For others, you will need to stretch your hymen in order to make an opening big enough for a penis (or even a tampon). If your hymen is thick and you don't stretch it out, and you and your husband decide to push through it on your wedding night, it will rip your hymen. This will cause a lot of pain, bleeding, and discomfort.

There are two things to remember about your hymen: it's important to know what your hymen looks like, and there are simple, easy ways to stretch your hymen without tearing it. I'll discuss these in Chapter 5.

Male Anatomy

On my wedding night, I kept thinking, "The only penis I've ever seen is Michaelangelo's David. Is this what they actually look like?"

—Lily

Because both men and women are created in the image of God, and because of the significance of gender in God's design for sex, it will be important for you to have a basic understanding of male anatomy. As awkward or unnecessary as it may seem, take some time to familiarize yourself with the male body with the help of scientific books, classes, websites, or a well-informed friend. Below, you'll find a basic overview of the male reproductive system and surrounding organs.

When you look at the area between a man's legs, you'll notice that many of his reproductive organs are located on the outside of his body. The most obvious organ is the penis, which is cylindrical in shape and several inches long, out of the tip of which comes both urine and semen. Similar to a woman's body, the skin covering his pubic area and surrounding the base of the penis is covered in pubic hair. Below the penis hangs the scrotum, a sac which contains two walnut-shaped testes, where all the sperm (male reproductive cells) is originally produced. Behind the scrotum is the anus, where poop comes out.

Okay, so let's break it down. Inside the scrotum are the testes, which produce millions and millions of sperm. This sperm travels out of the testes in a convoluted series of tubes that connect to the seminal gland. The seminal gland, along with several other glands, produce semen and other fluids that surround and support the sperm in its journey to an egg.

The seminal gland connects to the urethra, a tube running from the bladder to the exterior of the penis. That means both urine and semen flow through the urethra. During ejaculation, a sphincter closes off the opening to the bladder so no urine contaminates the semen, and during urination the semen is closed off so as not to contaminate the urine.

During sexual arousal, the penis, which is made up of muscles and blood vessels, hardens and enlarges until it becomes erect and about five to six inches long. This enables it to penetrate a vagina. At the peak of sexual arousal, the semen ejaculates out of the end of the penis, through the vagina, into the uterus, and up into a fallopian tube where it can connect with a woman's egg in order to form a zygote, the beginnings of a baby.

Knowing Your Body

*Once, I took a mirror and looked at myself just to see what it
looked like because I'd only seen illustrations. That helped me
realize that it's just part of me like my fingers and toes.*

—Ava

In the past, I never thought of women's sexual anatomy as having a lot
of variety. If someone had asked me, I might have said that all hymens
were the same. But some women are blond, some are brunette, some
are short and thin, some are tall and broad. So it stands to reason that
God would create the appearance and particulars of our sex organs
with variety as well.

During an interview with Dr. Cheryl Fogarty, OB/GYN, I asked what
every woman should know about her own anatomy. Dr. Fogarty's advice
was as enlightening as it was surprising: "I think you need to get
comfortable with yourself naked. Know what you have. Feel yourself.
Feel up inside. Know your size, your shape. A little knowledge goes a
long, long way."

This may be a shocking thing to hear. After all, many of us grew up
hearing things like, "Don't touch yourself," and most of us were taught
to use a cloth when it was time to wash "down there." So it seems crazy
to use your finger to feel yourself, especially up inside yourself, to know
your own anatomy. But we use our fingers to wipe our eyes and clean
out our fingernails and rub lotion on our elbows. Shouldn't we use our
hands to take care of, clean, and know our vaginas?

Here's a little tip: get a large, flat mirror and place it on the ground.
Lock the door, get naked, and stand over the mirror. (Sometimes it's
easier to prop the mirror on the wall, then squat or sit down, leaning
back.) Now spend some time looking at yourself. Identify your vulva,
your labia majora, your labia minora, your clitoris, and the clitoral hood.
Find your urethra, your vaginal opening, and your anus.

[handwritten: Did you?]

? Now, squat down a bit, peel back your labia, and look up your vagina. Can you see your hymen? If you can't see it, use your fingers to reach in and feel it. Is your hymen thick or thin? What's its shape? Crescent? All the way across with a small slit? Seemingly nonexistent?

Now stick your finger further up and discover your vagina. What's its shape? What does it feel like? Soft or firm? Smooth or rippled? How long is it? Four inches? Five? Two? How wide? Can you fit more than one finger?

[handwritten margin note: that would be dum]

Stick your finger up as far as you can and see if you can feel your cervix. Remember that your vagina is anywhere from two to four inches long, so you may have to reach pretty far with your finger in order to feel your cervix. The cervix is found at the end of your vagina (it's the "Do Not Enter" gate for your uterus), so once you feel the end of your vagina, you know you've found your cervix.

Depending on the time of your cycle, the end of your vagina (the cervix) may feel firm or soft, and it may be flat or stick out like a small, upside-down hill with a small opening at the top.

Now, back on the outside, find your clitoris again. Can you see it? Some women can and some can't. Remember, it's small and round, like the tip of your finger, surrounded by a "hood" at the point where your labia minora come together at the top. If you touch your clitoris, it will be very sensitive. One touch of your finger may send "zingers" through your body. At different times in your cycle, it may be swollen and big or perhaps small and hidden. *[handwritten: Period Sex]*

So there. Now you know your body a little better! What do you think? Did anything surprise you? What's your body like, and how is it different from the diagrams you've seen? Was it scary or did it feel weird to touch yourself and feel what was on the inside? Why do you think you felt this way?

Use your answers to these questions to understand yourself and your body better than you ever have before.

Your Cycle

I love being able to know where in my cycle I am, how to
manage my emotions with the time of month, and how to take
the time each month to care for myself. We, as women, need to
be familiar with our reproductive system, be in tune with our
cycle, and know how to truly care for ourselves, no matter
what age!

—Isabelle

I remember the day I got my period for the first time. I looked at my reflection in a mirror in total consternation and thought, "This is my life now? One fourth of my life is going to be like this?" But what I didn't realize is that my body is always on a loop, not one-fourth of the time, but all the time!

Each month (give or take a few days, depending on the person) your body preps eggs in your ovaries, then produces one egg (occasionally two) and sends it through your fallopian tubes to your uterus, where it then dies and your uterus sheds its lining, causing menstruation. (The only time this cycle alters is when the egg meets with a sperm and implants to produce a pregnancy.)

Once menstruation ends, it all starts again—prep eggs, send out one egg, egg dies, uterus sheds lining . . .

One day while on a walk, I realized that what my body goes through each month is a lot like the seasons that our world undergoes each year. Spring is the time before ovulation when your body "grows" the eggs. Summer is ovulation, when one egg bursts from your ovary, full of life. Autumn is menstruation, shedding the old lining of your uterus like colorful leaves. And winter is the dry time after your period when your body rests before doing it all over again.

You may find it helpful and interesting to recognize the signs of your cycle so that you can understand the seasons of your body.

Ovulation

The best way to determine when you ovulate is to observe the fluid present in your vagina. Whenever your body prepares to ovulate, your cervix creates a liquid that changes its consistency in the days before and after ovulation. Depending on what the liquid looks like, you can gauge how close you are to ovulating. You probably know what I'm talking about. When you wipe, it may feel super slippery. Or perhaps you notice a blob on your panties. Don't panic, this is just your cervical fluid.

In the days leading up to ovulation, the fluid will first be sticky or rubbery. After a couple days of this, it will turn creamy—like lotion—and might even be white. Next, the cervical fluid will turn into something that can only be described as egg-white. At this point, you are extremely fertile and will ovulate within a matter of days. Once you ovulate, your fluid will change back to creamy or sticky and then dry up completely.

If you want to observe your own cycle, start running your fingers across the opening of your vagina each day before you go to the bathroom. (Make sure to wash your hands first.) Feel and observe the fluid between your fingers and determine whether it's sticky, rubbery, creamy, or egg-whitish. (Your vagina is always a little wet, but if the substance dries on your fingers in a few seconds, then it's not cervical fluid, but the natural wetness of your vagina. This would be a "dry" vagina.)

If you observe your cervical fluid in this way for a couple months, you'll start to recognize your own natural cycle and know approximately when you ovulate each month.

In case you're wondering, if your vagina is "dry" and you don't have any cervical fluid, that means that you're not fertile. It's impossible to get pregnant when you're not ovulating, and you don't ovulate without producing cervical fluid. However, this process is way more nuanced than I've made it seem, and if you want to depend on natural methods for birth control or to plan a pregnancy, do your research. There are many helpful books, tools, and apps that help you determine the exact days of ovulation.

Menstruation

Menstruation occurs about twelve to fifteen days after ovulation, once your body is absolutely sure you're not pregnant. At this point, your uterus sheds the lining it has built up to prepare for pregnancy, and the blood and tissue pass through the cervix and out the vaginal opening.

For most women, menstruation lasts from three to five days, although anywhere from two to seven days is normal. The amount of menstrual fluid passed is different from woman to woman, but over the course of the period, most women pass about two and half tablespoons of fluid. (Anywhere between one and six tablespoons is considered normal.)

Even though it's often referred to as blood, menstrual fluid is only about 50% blood, the rest being a mixture of tissue and liquids from the uterus, cervix, and vagina. This menstrual fluid is completely clean and harmless. Remember, this is the same substance that nourishes a baby in the womb, so it's as pure as the blood in your veins! Sometimes blood clotting may occur, and it's easy to mistake these clots as tissue. When this happens, many women worry that they've had a miscarriage, but it is only the natural clotting of your blood.

Your period is controlled by hormones in your body, and in the days leading up to your period, these rising hormones may cause side effects such as acne, tender breasts, bloating, fatigue and irritability, and mood changes.

During your period, the heightened hormones may cause these same symptoms, as well as water retention, headaches, nausea, or a low sex drive. Many women also experience muscle cramping due to the shedding of the uterine wall lining.

Most women have their first period between the ages of twelve and fifteen, but it's normal to start as early as eight years old. This is called menarch. Menstruation continues to occur every month for the next several decades, until it gradually tapers off and ends completely. This is called menopause and generally occurs for most women between the ages of forty-five and fifty-five.

Becoming familiar with the interworking of your body can produce a huge appreciation for the beauty of the female body. Imagine the strength your body possesses to go through such huge changes on a regular basis. And it performs these arduous tasks all while you go on with your life– laughing, talking, working, and playing–carrying within yourself the mechanism of life itself. How awesome is it that women's bodies are always ready to create life?

Praise God for Yourself

Men go abroad to wonder at the height of mountains, at the huge waves of the sea, at the long courses of the rivers, at the vast compass of the ocean, at the circular motion of the stars; and they pass by themselves without wondering.
–Saint Augustine

A key element of having a godly sexuality is to understand your identity as one of God's creations. One of the most life-changing experiences I've ever had has to do with this concept of seeing yourself through the eyes of your Creator.

One day I met with my mentor to talk and pray together. While praying, I started praising God for his creation and for how beautiful it is. But when I was done, my mentor said, "You love to praise God about his creation, but you don't praise him for his most wonderful creation– you!"

Her words weren't Hallmark-card fluff. They were sound doctrine concerning the nature of humanity. God made man and woman and said that it was very good.

So one day I went into my room, took a piece of paper and a pen, and wrote a psalm of praise to God for myself. It was so weird to think of my body and my personality and my quirks, not from a personal standpoint, as though they were my own, but looking at myself as an original piece of art made by God's own hands. I couldn't hate my short legs or the fact that my eyes aren't big. Instead, I praised him for my cute, tiny shins and my almond-shaped eyes. I praised him for my hair, my big cheeks, and the way my eyes crinkle when I smile. I praised him that I like to learn and to encourage people and that I require inordinate amounts of sleep every day.

This activity has completely changed the way I view myself. I've learned to look even at my body not as my own but as God's creation. When I think of myself not as my own but as someone created by God for his glory, it drastically alters my point of view when it comes to how I care for, use, and think about my body.

I challenge you to write your own psalm of praise to God for your body and personality and sexuality. Praise him for both the things you love and the things you hate about yourself. Praise him for your gender, for the potential your female body has to have sex and to have children. Praise him for sexual desire, both as a means of developing patience and intimacy with God when you're single and as a way to experience intimacy with a man when you're married. Use your imagination to think of how God must see you and everything that makes up "you" since he is the one who created you. Let this reshape your understanding of yourself, your body, and your sexuality.

3

Caring for Your Body

When you truly believe that your body and health is a gift from God and you work at being a good steward of that gift, you will value your womanhood and have such a positive self-worth!
—Chloe

Don't you realize that your body is the temple of the Holy Spirit, who lives in you and was given to you by God? You do not belong to yourself, for God bought you with a high price. So you must honor God with your body.
—1 Corinthians 6:19–20 NLT

Scripture mentions priests whose only job was to take care of the temple. They spent their time sweeping the floors, trimming the candle wicks, and brushing ash off the altar. And the name by which these actions were known? Worship. Taking care of the temple was worship, no matter how mundane it must have felt for them to push that broom across the floor. It was worship, and it was a way to honor God.

And then, in the New Testament, Paul says that our bodies are God's new temple. Taking care of your body is a form of worship, a way of honoring God. He's the one who made your body and he has a purpose for it, so you should treat it like the heavenly gift that it is, no matter how mundane it may feel to wash your face, trim your nails, and brush your hair. Paul goes so far as to say that God bought your body, so it's not even yours anymore to decide what to do with it! So honor God with your body.

Basic Self Care

I'd wanted to hide my sexuality for so long it felt unnatural to learn to care for myself, but I've been released from that shame and now it's just part of a daily routine. I enjoy finding out new ways to care for myself through talking with my girlfriends about what they do and being honest with them about my struggles and questions.

—Alice

There are all kinds of ways to take care of your body on a regular basis. Here is a list of things you should do:

- Wash your face with a gentle cleanser daily.
- Wash your hair every 1-3 days.
- Wash your body every 1-3 days.
- Brush, floss, and rinse your teeth twice daily.
- Clean and dry your vulva daily.
- Clean and trim your fingernails and toenails as needed.
- Clean your ears every 1-3 days. (Be careful if you use Q-tips, as it can be incredibly dangerous for your eardrums if a Q-tip is inserted too far into your ear canal.)
- Moisturize your face, body, hands, hair, and lips with lotion or oil as needed.

Cleaning Your Vagina   *Smell*

> The robust vagina is an acidic vagina, with a pH of 3.8 to 4.5.
> That's somewhat more acidic than black coffee (with a pH of 5)
> but less piquant than a lemon (pH 2). In fact, the idea of pairing
> wine and women isn't a bad one, as the acidity of the vagina in
> health is just about that of a glass of red wine.
> —Natalie Angier

Did you know that your vagina is pH balanced? This means that both yeast and bacteria are present, existing in a perfectly balanced state so that your vagina is clean and works correctly.

You may have heard someone refer to a woman's smell as "fishy," but if a woman's vagina smells fishy, that means she has an infection. To help your vagina stay clean and balanced, wash with plain, clean water. If you use harsh soaps or douches, this will chemically alter the environment of your vagina and will almost certainly introduce infection.

In the shower, simply open your labia and let water flow over your vagina. Or a good soak in the bathtub will do the trick. Some women like to fill a squirt bottle with warm water and squirt around their vagina, especially during their periods, to keep clean. If you do use a soap, choose something mild and pH balanced and never wash inside your vagina, only around your vulva and inside your labia majora and labia minora.

However, it may seem like for all the talk about keeping your vagina pH balanced, there's still a strong odor coming from your vagina even when you don't have an infection. This is because there are sweat glands all around the vaginal opening. Just as your armpits stink when you sweat, your vagina will stink if it sweats and is kept warm and moist under tight clothing. Here are three suggestions for preventing odor:

No Panties at Night ⱱ̣ᴏᵛ

Imagine a typical day in which you wear panties all day, maybe work out, then come home and sit down to eat without changing. It's easy to see how a hot and sweaty environment like this would make your vagina stink! But if you sleep without panties every night, you'll allow your genitals to air-dry and cool, thus preventing the bacteria that flourishes in warm, moist environments.

No Sweaty Clothes

Change out of your workout clothes immediately after exercising. Dr. Fogarty suggests putting on a pair of loose cotton shorts, without any underwear, to air-dry after exercising.

Wear Cotton Underwear

Cotton allows the most airflow of any fabric, so it will best keep your vagina cool and dry. Remember, it's when things are warm and damp that bacteria and yeast grow.

Pubic Hair

I have given up trying to keep myself totally bare. Although that would be lovely, it's just not worth the itch, don't you agree? I just shave around making a triangle that fits within a bikini. I also cut the hair, so it's shorter.
—Evelyn

There is a wide range of opinion and practice when it comes to dealing with the hair on your vulva. Most of it is a matter of opinion and preference, so take your pick!

Trimmed

Buy a pair of those little kid scissors in the school supplies section. They're small and easy to maneuver and have blunt ends. Cut your pubic hair down as short as you comfortably can with a pair of these scissors. I recommend trimming your hair while sitting on the toilet, because this will be the most convenient position with which to see your vaginal area and you can simply flush all the hair down the toilet when you're done. If some of your hair grows outside your bikini zone (i.e., if you can see it even when you're wearing underwear), take some shaving cream and a razor and shave that section completely off. This is the practice that Dr. Fogarty recommends. She states that it will discourage infection and promote cleanliness if nothing can cling to your pubic hair.

Shaved

My friend Hannah has written great step-by-step instructions for those of you wanting to shave everything:

> Trim your pubic hair, with scissors, as short as you possibly can. Soak your skin in warm/hot water for at least five minutes. I do this when I take showers or baths.

> After about five minutes, lather up some nice shaving cream or soap (shaving cream is best but soap will work). Let the soap or shaving cream set on your skin for about 1–2 minutes. Then, slowly and softly, shave upward on your skin. I try to use nice razors, not the real cheap ones, if possible.

> After you have shaved, wash off the remaining soap or shaving cream. Dry off your skin with a towel and then apply baby powder. Baby powder seems to help me even more than lotion.

If you choose to shave everything, stay consistent! In fact, never go more than two to three days without shaving. There are two reasons for this. One, as your hair grows out, it gets incredibly itchy. (It's basically

29

torture.) Two, the more you shave, the easier and faster it becomes. Before long, you'll be able to shave yourself in only a minute or two.

Waxed

If you wish to wax your bikini area or even your entire vaginal area (called a Brazilian wax), I recommend going to a professional. Most salons and spas offer this service.

You will be shown into a private room with a massage or examination table. The technician will apply a strip of warm wax on a section of the hair, then press a piece of treated paper to the wax. After a few moments the wax begins to harden, adhering to both the hair and the paper. Firmly grasping an edge of the paper, the technician will rip off the wax in a swift, strong movement, removing the hair with it.

This process can be painful, but applying pressure, ice, or soothing creams can alleviate some of the pain.

Your hair must be at least a quarter inch long to wax. Once the hair has been removed, growth does not occur for many days and most women only need to wax every three to four weeks.

Untrimmed

Even though my gynecologist does not recommend this, I have to add it for a number of reasons. First, it's possible to keep your pubic hair clean even if it is long. Secondly, it's become so trendy to completely remove the hair from the vaginal area that a friend of mine recently told me all of her teenage daughter's friends shave their vulvas!

Even though each woman has every right to do what she wants with her pubic hair, I don't think any woman should ever be expected to completely shave or wax her hair. A woman's body is meant to have pubic hair, and I would hate to get to the place in our culture where pubic hair is considered unfeminine or not "sexy." As a good friend and college biology professor likes to say, "We are mammals, after all!"

Infection

I have struggled with yeast infections since junior high. So it
flares up now and then.
                                        —Ruby

While there are many different types of infection that a woman may encounter, here we'll focus on two infections related to female sexual anatomy: urinary tract infection (UTI) and vaginal yeast infection.

Urinary Tract Infection

One night in my early twenties, I kept waking up feeling like I had to go to the bathroom. I probably was up more than ten times that night, but little to no urine would come out. There was no specific area of pain, but I felt extremely uncomfortable and had a burning sensation when I tried to pee. The next morning I made a doctor's appointment, and she easily diagnosed it as a UTI.

Some symptoms of a UTI are: burning or pain when you pee, a strong urge to urinate, lower abdominal or vaginal pain, lower back pain, blood in the urine or on toilet paper when you wipe, fever, and chills.

If you think you may have a UTI, there are many home remedies that can fight the infection. Drink plenty of water (until you're urinating every thirty to sixty minutes) to flush the infection from your system, drink cranberry juice to add acidity to your system that may help restore the pH balance of your body, cut out sugar and dairy which both feed bacteria, and eat lots of yogurt or take a probiotic. If you do this, as well as maintain a clean, dry vaginal area and continue to wipe yourself from front to back, the infection may go away on its own.

If you're doing these things and still feel bad after twenty-four hours, make a doctor's appointment. A UTI can easily travel up your urinary tract and become a bladder or a kidney infection if it gets too bad. A doctor will prescribe an antibiotic that will quickly clear up the infection and get you feeling better soon. (If you have lower back pain, fever, or blood in your urine, see a doctor immediately.)

Vaginal Yeast Infection

This infection occurs when there is an overgrowth of yeast in the vagina. It's so common that 75 percent of women report having at least one in their lifetime.[8] Symptoms include intense itching in the vaginal or vulva, burning sensation while urinating, vaginal discharge (either a water-like discharge or a thick, white, odorless discharge), and irritation on the vagina or vulva.

Vaginal yeast infections can be caused by antibiotic use (the antibiotics kill the naturally occurring bacteria in your body that holds the yeast at bay), a suppressed immune system (i.e., injury or chemotherapy), pregnancy, oral contraceptives, and douches.

Vaginal yeast infections are easily treated with prescription anti-fungal medication, over-the-counter yeast infection medications, or natural remedies such as coconut oil and yogurt (applied topically, these things have been known to treat yeast infections in some cases).

You can prevent yeast infections by cleaning yourself from front to back and avoiding chemicals and things that may upset the pH balance of your vagina, such as douches, scented tampons and dryer sheets, and unnecessary antibiotics. Eating yogurt and drinking lots of water can also help prevent yeast infections.

Medical Exam

I think it's important to find an OB/GYN with whom you feel
comfortable asking any question. If the doctor makes you feel
dumb, uncomfortable, or rushed, find another doctor.
                                    —Lucy

It's recommended that every woman have regular checkups with an OB/GYN (that stands for obstetrician and gynecologist). Make an appointment for a date when you are not menstruating. Before going to the doctor, clean your genitals with water or with a wet wipe. You may also wish to jot down any questions you have regarding your sexual health (i.e., "Is my vagina healthy?" "What can I do to prevent infection?" "Is it normal for...?").

You should know that an exam by an OB/GYN is not the most fun thing in the world. You usually start by peeing into a cup. (In case you ever wondered, you only have to fill up the cup about a third of the way.) Once in the examination room, you'll be asked some questions about your health and sexual activity. You'll be asked to undress and be given a medical gown. Take off everything, including your bra and panties, although you can leave your socks on if you wish.

Later, the doctor will come in to conduct the exam. You'll be instructed to lie on your back on the examination table, lift your knees, and place your feet in stirrups so that the doctor can properly view your vagina. The doctor will use her or his fingers and hands to examine the inside of your vagina. The doctor will also swab the cells of your cervix in order to check for infection or disease. This is called a pap smear.

Sometimes, in order to do a pap smear, the doctor will insert a speculum into your vagina. A speculum is a metal device that looks much like a curling iron. The doctor will insert it, then slowly open it until your vagina stretches enough to examine your vagina and take a

terrifying
but ok

No it doesn't

33

more uncomfortable than anything

sample. This stretching may cause a burning or painful sensation, but it will only last a few moments.

The doctor will also use his or her hands to give you a breast exam and to press on your abdomen as a way to check on your internal organs.

After the exam is a good time to ask any questions you may have. Go back for an exam and pap smear once a year with your OB/GYN.

Keeping Clean During Your Cycle

I take more showers and keep myself very clean while on my period. Cleanliness has helped me feel more comfortable.
—Maya

There are several things you can do to keep clean during your cycle. Always wipe from front to back, and keep your genitals clean and dry. During times when you're bleeding or have vaginal discharge, you have many different options for keeping your genitals and clothes clean.

Pads

The most common option is to wear a pad or panty liner on your underwear to catch the blood or fluid. If you use a pad, replace it every two to four hours. Never flush a pad, but instead remove it and wrap it in toilet paper before disposing of it in the trash. Pads and panty liners are easy to use and easy to find. One disadvantage is that blood sometimes leaks onto your panties or clothing. Also, scented pads can cause irritation on sensitive skin.

Tampons

Another common method is to wear a tampon, a tube made of cotton inserted into your vagina, where it soaks up the blood before it even comes out.

Change tampons every two to four hours. Make sure that you insert the applicator fully into your vagina before pushing the tampon out of the applicator and further into your vagina. An attached string will hang out of your vagina for easy removal. Never flush a tampon. Instead, remove the tampon and wrap it in toilet paper before throwing it in the trash.

Tampons are a popular option because they absorb a lot of blood, have less leakage, aren't as bulky as a pad, and, used in conjunction with a pad, can do "double duty" on heavy days or nights. Some women find that they can't use tampons if their vagina is too narrow or if their hymen covers the opening of their vagina. Also, tampons can cause irritation or infection, especially if they are scented or made with chemicals. Another disadvantage is that they often still require the use of a pad or panty liner to catch any leakage.

Menstrual Cup

Another option is something called a menstrual cup. A menstrual cup is a small, silicone "cup" about two inches long that is inserted into your vagina, much like a tampon, but instead of absorbing the blood, it catches it. When it's full, you simply remove the cup and dump the contents into the toilet, wash the cup with soap and warm water, and put it back in.

Many women like this option because it's reusable and thus cheaper, has less leakage, is clean and hypoallergenic, only needs to be emptied twice a day, and lends itself to an increased familiarity with your body and your blood flow. Some cons associated with a menstrual cup are that it is not as widely available, is difficult to use in public restrooms, takes practice to insert correctly, and requires knowledge and familiarity with your body.

Although you'll learn to go about your life during your period, it may help to be easy on your body during this time. Take a nap. Take ibuprofen. Perhaps you choose to stay away from people when you're moody. A heating pad can do wonders for cramps. Drink a little caffeine to get rid of a headache caused by hormones. Remember all the hard work your body is doing and give it grace to get the job done.

Kegel Exercises

After I started having sex, it's like all my muscles down there just went kaput. I had almost zero bladder control and started having accidents. Like a two-year-old. Once, I wet the bed right next to my new husband! He just stared at me with this look of pity mixed with amusement and then sweetly helped me change the sheets in the middle of the night. I started doing Kegel exercises shortly after, to strengthen my muscles down there.

—Thea

Kegel exercises are one type of exercise that is extremely important for women's sexual health. They are done to tone up and work out the muscles in your vagina. The next time you go to the bathroom, try to stop your pee mid-flow. In other words, pee, then stop. Then pee a little more, then stop. The muscles that you're using to perform this action are the muscles in your pelvic floor. Once you recognize what it feels like to use these muscles, you can flex and relax them anytime you want. When you flex and relax these muscles, you're performing a Kegel exercise.

You can perform Kegel exercises two different ways. The first way is a slow Kegel exercise, and to do this you tighten the muscles of your pelvic floor and hold for three seconds. Relax your muscles and then repeat. The second way is a fast Kegel exercise, and you do this by tightening and relaxing your muscles as quickly as you can. Practice either exercise until you can perform them easily and up to fifty times. Do this daily.

Performing Kegels will keep your vagina strong and healthy and, later in life, will help you in childbirth, during sex, and when dealing with bladder incontinence in your old age.

* important

4

How to Be a Darling When You're Single

I wish someone had told me that I would grow into my sexuality. That I would feel freedom and confidence with time, we both would. It's okay for it to take time. It can take years, decades even. The journey is not one to be rushed; it's one to enjoy.

—Millie

As Christian women, we've been told to keep our innocence when it comes to sex, but we've also been kept ignorant, often until the very moment we walk down the aisle.

—Mattie

= Shawna?
1- huge prob.

With an understanding of God's design for sex, as well as of your own body, you will be on solid footing as you move forward in the discovery of your sexuality.

What's crazy is now that we know sexuality is a picture of our relationships with Jesus Christ, we see that it can also be expressed in singleness. Being chaste (having godly sexuality) means nothing more than using your sexuality to express the relationship between Christ and his church. So, if you're single or dating, that means that you can be chaste by abstaining from sex, while simultaneously embracing your sexuality and the longing you feel.

As a single person, you may be longing to find someone, to be married, or to have sex. It's a very palpable, visceral feeling within you. That's the kind of longing that Christians should have for the coming of Jesus! Not only that, but that's the kind of longing we all should feel to experience union with Jesus right now.

Single people play such an important role in the church! We need you to display for us what it means to live with a desire not yet satisfied. We need your example of holy longing mixed with patient faith.

very rough

While married people can teach the church what it means to enter into covenant unity with God, this is something that can't be fully realized until heaven. The picture that single people provide is a realistic portrait of what the life of the believer is like—a longing for Jesus in the midst of a painful struggle.

In this chapter, we'll discuss what it means to be a darling as a single woman and present some ideas for living a life of chastity.

Affirming the Goodness of Sex

> *It took me awhile to realize how I was inadvertently insulting God by my hesitation to accept the holiness of sex and pleasure. I don't have any problem imagining someone seeking God by enduring the pain of a fast. But what kind of God am I imagining if I can allow pain but not pleasure to reveal God's presence in my life?* interesting
> —*Gary Thomas*

Because sex was created by God, a big part of having godly sexuality is to acknowledge that sex is good. It's not sinful, dirty, or weird when used in accordance with God's plan; it is good, pure, and beautiful—a true gift. Whether you are single or dating, you must fight the urge to criticize or ignore your sexuality in an effort to stay pure. Remember, a large part of purity is thinking about sex the way God does!

Be Aware of Your Sexuality

Do you ever feel warm and tingly when a man you like smiles in your direction? That's a sexual experience. Have you ever experienced a pleasant sensation, centered around your vulva, while in a warm shower or snuggled in bed? That's a sexual experience. Have you ever watched a movie that leaves your heart beating and your panties a little wet? That's a sexual experience. God created you to have these experiences. It's not a sin to be turned on, but rather a natural part of being human. Sexual sin occurs when you step outside of God's guidelines for sex. For example, while you have no control over feeling warm and tingly when a man smiles at you, you must not lust (imagining and desiring sex with someone you're not married to). Fornication (having sex before marriage) and adultery (having sex with someone who is married) are two other forms of sexual sin. Recognize the difference between a natural expression of your sexuality and sexual sin.

Thank God for Your Sexuality

One healthy way of processing your sexuality or a sexual experience (feeling turned on, being tempted to lust, etc.) is to thank God that you have these feelings. Your sexuality is what will enable you, once married, to participate in the intimacy of sexual union, an amazing experience so unrivaled that it's a reminder of intimacy with the Almighty God! Your sexuality is a sacred charge, an enormous responsibility, and at times a burden that you bear so that you can glorify God in your obedience, submission, and later, during marriage, through your enjoyment of his good gift.

Turn to God for Satisfaction

When a man and a woman come together during sex and become one person, this represents something beautiful about the nature of the Trinity and the intimate communion that God is inviting you into. However, God offers the real deal—an invitation into the community of the Trinity—to every believer, wedded or not. One woman I interviewed says it this way: "Only God can satisfy. Sex is just like everything else in life—eventually it will leave you unfulfilled, no matter how good it is." Similarly, The Message Bible paraphrases Jonah 2:8 by saying, "Those who worship hollow gods, god-frauds, walk away from their only true love." Sex is a shadow of the relationship that is already available to you. Whoever you are, whatever stage in life you're in, turn to God, your one true love.

Abstaining from Sex

The unmarried Christian who practices chastity refrains from sex in order to remember that God desires your person, your body, more than any man or woman ever will.
                    —Lauren F. Winner

Good reminder for me.

Because sex was meant to be experienced in the context of marriage, being a single or dating woman will mean refraining from sexual activity with yourself and others. You honor God's plan by engaging in sexuality the way he intended, even if that means not engaging in sex at all. Here we'll discuss fornication, masturbation, same-sex attraction, and sexual abuse, four areas of sexual activity that go against God's plan for those he deeply loves.

Fornication

So easy no matter how strong.

Fornication is having sex without being married, and it is not a part of God's plan for sex. But in a heated, lonely moment with your boyfriend, vague verses from the Bible hardly keep you level-headed. So . . . what actually helps? How can you remain chaste when you are dating? Here are a few ideas:

1. Confession

Confession is an incredibly practical and effective tool against sin in a believer's life. It's easy for your personal sin to seem inconsequential when it stays in your head and in the privacy of a dark basement, but when you're sitting across from another Christian, saying words like masturbation, pornography, and oral sex, it's not so easy to feel justified. Plus, there's a sense in which confession works almost like magic—"If we confess our sins, he is faithful and just to forgive us our sins and to cleanse us from all unrighteousness" (1 John 1:9 ESV). Just try it and see.

2. Boundaries

If you do set limits on your sexual activity, make sure you consider your personal weakness, history, and personality, as well as those of your boyfriend. And make them with the help of another Christian (or two) who know you both well. Some people may be able to make out with passion and affection, then continue watching their movie while gently holding hands. Another couple may not even trust themselves to be alone together. Rules won't save you, but don't be foolish. Proper boundaries can go a long way in your journey of sexual purity.[9]

3. Just Say No

I rarely say no to myself. The trouble is, I have lots of self-destructive urges. I want three cups of coffee every morning. I want to eat chips every night while I watch TV. I want my husband to spend every moment at home playing with my hair while looking deeply into my eyes and making interesting conversation (just kidding . . . sort of).

Once I started paying attention to the moments when my desires were self-destructive, I felt shocked by how often I needed to say no to myself. In fact, it was kind of overwhelming and depressing. But it's given me a very rooted awareness of my own sinfulness, my inability even to want to do what's right, and my need for the righteousness of Jesus. Now, as Jesus does the work of making me new from the inside out, I am realizing the validity of saying no to myself.

I also remind myself that every time I say no to myself, I'm saying yes to something else. The decision to kill your desires sets you free to become the person you want to be. You may have to say no to your sexual urges sometimes, but by the grace of God and through the help of the Holy Spirit, you're saying yes to the chaste, fulfilling and fruitful life of a darling.

Masturbation

Masturbation is when you stimulate yourself using your hand, fingers, an object, or a sex toy (such as a vibrator) in order to feel sexual pleasure, and it usually ends in orgasm. This practice is generally approved of in our culture, and according to the National Survey of Sexual Health and Behavior, most adult women have masturbated at least once.[10]

The Bible never directly addresses the issue of masturbation, so we have to apply general principles of God's character and wisdom in order to discern what is best.

My personal opinion is that masturbation is not a part of godly sexuality. Here's my reasoning—sex is meant to be between two people for the ultimate purpose of intimacy and the glory of God. While there may be dozens of reasons why a woman would choose to masturbate, it's hard for me to find any that completely fulfill this God-given purpose of sex.

However, there are many faithful Christians who believe differently. Even Christian counselors and therapists sometimes recommend masturbation for those who are single, for those in marriages with a spouse with a low sex drive, for men who need to practice lasting longer during sex, or for women who are learning to be more orgasmic. As mentioned before, the Bible does not address the issue of masturbation, so I give full grace to my Christian brothers and sisters who engage in the practice of masturbation as a means of promoting sexual purity or better intimacy in marriage. (Please understand, this does not condone the practice of masturbation when accompanied by lust or pornography or in the company of someone to whom you are not married.)

My suggestion is spend some time studying and praying in order to decide for yourself what you believe about masturbation. Then seek God and other believers' help in acting upon that belief in a way that honors him. *personal decision, but how can you w/out lusting?*

Same-Sex Attraction

People who are same-sex attracted feel sexually attracted to members of the same gender. While this goes against God's design for sex (sex is between a man and a woman), know that the feelings themselves are not sinful, but only lustful thoughts and homosexual acts. Whatever your background or current experience, if you have feelings of same-sex attraction, here are a couple of things that I'd love for you to know:

1. You Are Not Alone
Sometimes feelings of same-sex attraction can leave you feeling like an outsider, like no one knows how you feel. But there are many men and women who experience similar feelings, and many of them are Christians. You're not the only one to feel this way, and there are people who have walked this road ahead of you.

But more than that, God is walking this road with you. God loves people who are same-sex attracted. God loves you fully and faithfully. He wants to have a relationship with you and to invite you into his family. You don't have to be alone.

2. It's Good to Tell Someone

If you have feelings of same-sex attraction, tell a trusted Christian friend. It can be incredibly isolating to hide these feelings, and you may fear the reaction of those around you. But when you let yourself be vulnerable about this aspect of your life, you open yourself up to receive the love and safety of Christ's love for you through the church. This love often comes in the form of deep and lasting friendships, full of the intimacy that we all crave.

Every Christian is broken and has to fight against feelings and temptations that lead us away from God's plan for us. Being honest with yourself and your closest friends can not only lift a heavy burden from your shoulders but also be an encouragement to your friends as they live with their own brokenness. When we are honest about our problems, then we open ourselves up both to receive and to give help.

3. Your Identity Comes from Your Creator

Many people choose to place their identity in their sexuality, saying things like "I'm gay" or "I'm straight." But for the Christian, we realize that our central identity comes from God, the creator and lover of our souls. We are not defined by our sexuality (or our race, background, achievements, etc.); we are defined by something much bigger, much more whole and dependable. Just because you have feelings of same-sex attraction doesn't mean that your identity has shifted unless you decide that it has.

My encouragement is to ground your identity in God alone. Nowhere else will you find such a faithful and robust love. God will never leave you nor forsake you. In him is satisfaction and joy and the salvation of your soul. Whatever you give up to get Jesus is totally worth it.

Sexual Abuse

Sex is a beautiful gift from God, but ever since the fall, humanity has been breaking God's gifts—all of creation—as a result of sin and our own brokenness. One of the most painful and horrifying results of sin is the presence of sexual abuse in the world.

Rape and inappropriate touching are often what we think of when we speak of sexual abuse, but it also involves much more than that. A basic definition of sexual abuse includes "any behavior, attitude, or verbal response that hinders normal sexual development, bringing distortion and inhibition to personal sexuality and married lovemaking."[11]

Sadly, there are too many different kinds of abuse to even list here, but it's important to remember that any unwanted sexual behavior forced on you is sexual abuse. This can mean anything from someone watching you undress, to someone exposing himself or herself in your presence, unwanted sex play with other children when you were younger, and rape or sexual touching. Any of this is abuse, whether it happens at the hand of a stranger, friend, family member, boyfriend, or husband.

If this has ever happened to you, no matter the circumstances, it was not your fault. After a confusing and painful experience like this, you may feel a heavy burden of guilt, but a victim is never responsible for sexual abuse.

An experience of sexual assault is both traumatizing and complex, and most people are not able to move forward without help. Thankfully, there are many resources for receiving help, whether your abuse was in the past or is currently taking place. Here are three ways to seek help and find healing:

1. Medical Care

If you have been raped, you can seek immediate medical attention. Go to the ER and let the medical professionals know what has happened so that they can provide you with the care you need and so that they can discover and preserve any evidence that will help with the conviction of the person who has hurt you. If your abuse was in the past, it would be wise to have an exam with a doctor who knows what has happened. The doctor will be able to check for any injuries or infections that may exist as a result.

2. Law Enforcement

If you have been abused, you can call 911. You are the victim of a heinous crime, and the abuser deserves punishment for his or her behavior. However, such action can feel overwhelming or frightening at a time like this. If so, know that you can call and report the incident without having to file a charge until you are ready. You may also request that law enforcement come to you at the ER or medical clinic for your privacy and safety.

3. Counseling

While sharing your story with a trusted friend or family member will be a first step, in the case of abuse a therapist will be an invaluable tool in processing what has happened and healthfully moving forward. Find a Christian counselor with specialized training in helping sexual abuse survivors. This will be an important relationship, so if you start meeting with the counselor and find that, after a couple of weeks, you don't "click," don't be afraid to find someone else. Also, if the counselor ever suggests that the abuse was your fault, find another counselor.

There is a conspiracy of silence surrounding sexual assault. It's very difficult for a survivor of sexual abuse to speak about her experience. There are many reasons that she may not want to tell anyone about what happened. These are natural feelings, but none of them should keep her from getting the help she needs and from the abuser receiving the consequences of his or her crime. If you are a survivor of sexual abuse, please start by telling a trusted friend or family member. Those who love you should stand beside you as you decide how to best move forward.

And finally, even though you bear no guilt as a victim of sexual abuse, you may have had to shoulder the crushing weight of shame as a result of what's happened to you. Merriam-Webster defines shame as "a painful emotion caused by consciousness of guilt, shortcoming, or impropriety."[12] However, in the case of sexual abuse, the victim has had an improper act forced upon her. So although she is not guilty, she may feel the shame of having been involved in such a humiliating and disgraceful act.

Amazingly, Jesus died on the cross to take away not only the guilt of sinners but also shame. "Christ loved the church and gave himself up for her to make her holy, cleansing her by the washing with water through the word, and to present her to himself as a radiant church, without stain or wrinkle or any other blemish, but holy and blameless" (Eph. 5:25–27 NIV). Jesus sees no stain or wrinkle on you. You are not "damaged goods" but instead have the purity and radiance of Jesus himself. Whatever has happened, however you are feeling, Jesus sees you as his beloved bride and has moved heaven and earth to keep you at his side.[13]

Overcoming Sexual Sin

*To break the habit [of masturbation] I would sit up in bed until
I was so exhausted I couldn't do it. I would hold my hands
above my head, sometimes holding the head board so I wasn't
tempted. I would read or watch TV until I fell asleep. It really
helped to understand the urges were normal and natural, but
that God intended those urges to bring intimacy with my
husband—not immediate, personal pleasure.*

          —Sienna

I started having crushes on boys when I was about seven years old.
These crushes quickly developed into elaborate fantasies that became
more and more sexual as I neared puberty. Once I was older and knew
myself better, I realized that I was dealing with issues of sexual purity,
and my own struggle with lust haunted me. Once I was in a serious
relationship, these fantasies became much more specific. Namely, I
thought about having sex with my boyfriend. I remember thinking, "If I
can just make it to marriage, all of this will disappear."

But marriage can't fix our sin—only Jesus can. Although my struggle
was very real, very sinful, and very overwhelming, I didn't have to live so
defeated. If I had taken my sin to the cross, understanding that his
death paid the punishment for my sin, I would've realized the extent of
God's love for me and the truth that sin no longer has power in my life.
Once I did, I found that it was out of this place of love and grace that
God could begin the work of changing my heart so that I could desire
what is good, not what is sinful.

If you struggle with sexual sin, spend time meditating on the cross.
Remember that you are already forgiven for every sin you have
committed in the past and every sin you will commit in the future. Jesus
takes your sexual impurity, suffers the punishment of a sexual offender,
and you walk away pure (see 2 Cor. 5:21). That is your status before God.
That is why the gospel is such good news. "While we were still sinners,

Christ died for us" (Rom. 5:8 NIV). Let this truth sink into your heart until it permeates your whole life.

Once you understand that even your sexual sin does not need to separate you from God, you can use these age-old tools to allow God to reshape your thinking about sexuality:

Read the Bible

Read a lot of it. Let the truth of God's word saturate your heart and your mind. I know this may sound demanding, but I challenge you to read the Bible until it dilutes the potency of all the magazines, social media, movies, TV, and relationships that often pour lies into your mind. Let the Bible be the biggest influence in your life. *so true*

Pray

After hearing God's Word, respond to him in prayer. He is your Father, and he wants to hear from you. Praise him for who he is, thank him for what he has done, confess your sins to him, and ask him for help to live a godly life. Feel the freedom to be completely honest with him, telling him about your struggles. "Give all your worries and cares to God, for he cares about you" (1 Pet. 5:7 NLT).

Find a Godly Community

It can be so disheartening if your friends disdain you for your virginity. In fact, it can make you feel embarrassed, which is the opposite of what God wants for you. But if you're around other women and men who value and treasure their own chastity as well as yours, you can feel safe enough to be who God wants you to be.

Find a Godly Mentor

You need someone whom you can talk to about your sexuality, someone to whom you can confess your sins and your shortcomings and your struggles, someone who will ask you about those weaknesses when you forget to or don't want to talk about them.

Find a Godly Counselor

Sometimes there are issues that your friends and mentors may not know how to handle. But counselors are trained professionals, and many Christian counselors are passionate about leading you out of harmful lies and into the truth of God's Word. Sometimes, if you're willing and eager to learn, a counselor's words can help you fix big problems. My husband often says, "Asking for help is a sign of strength." A counselor is especially helpful if you are dealing with issues of abuse, sexual addiction, homosexuality, or pornography.

Singleness and Intimacy

When I was single, I focused on my goals and what I wanted for my future. I didn't allow that season of my life to go by without doing things. I traveled, tried new hobbies and hung out with a variety of people. I wanted to do something incredible with my time. I knew that God was using me!

—Layla

Cameron Cole writes, "Your desire for sex really is a desire for deep connection with God and people. You do not have to wait until marriage to experience and enjoy intimacy. It is available for you here and now in your relationship with Christ and through vibrant friendships. Perhaps sex will be one of many ways that you enjoy intimacy at some point in your life. However, sex is only one way. Better options exist before and even after marriage."[14]

This kind of holistic approach to sexuality is essential to understanding that the true purpose of sexuality is intimacy. It helps us to place sexuality within the larger context of all the forms of intimacy that God has bestowed upon us.

While I'm not trying to say that our relationship with God or other people is sexual, I am suggesting that it's impossible to have a healthy view of sexuality if we don't understand its proper place in our lives—smack dab in the middle of all our other relationships.

Become aware of the people whom you connect with on a deep level. Nurture these friendships by spending time with these people, telling them how much they mean to you, showing your true self, and accepting their true selves in return. This will lead to the kinds of "vibrant friendships" that provide deeply satisfying intimacy in your life.

Pursue intimacy with God. Grow your friendship with God by reading the Bible, praying, obeying God's Word, and meditating on Jesus's enormous act of friendship toward you on the cross. This will lead to the deep levels of intimacy of which the psalmist spoke when he said, "Whom have I in heaven but you? And there is nothing on earth that I desire besides you" (Ps. 73:25 ESV).

God has made true intimacy available to each of his children. If you're single, you're not left out. God wants you to plumb the depths of intimacy, both with other people and ultimately with himself.

Part Two

Engaged Darlings

5

How to Be a Darling When You're Engaged

God is working in our waiting.
—Betsy Childs Howard

Engagement is really, really hard.
—Holly

[handwritten: But much harder]

For those of you engaged to be married, first of all, congratulations! This is an exciting time for you. If you're engaged, chastity will look much the same as when you're single or dating. In a spiritual sense, you're still single, not yet "joined together" with a man in marriage. Continue living life as a darling—knowing you are deeply loved by God—by abstaining from sex while still affirming its goodness.

However, as an engaged couple anxiously waiting for marriage, you can also act out your chastity during engagement through communicating as a couple about past and current sexual activity, by preparing for the sex you will have together in the future, and by learning how to "flip the switch."

[handwritten: So be careful your sexual activity before hand]

57

Communication

Be honest with each other! Be honest about your heart, your
fears, your struggles, your joys, your past, and your dreams for
the future. If you can't share it, then it won't get any easier and
you'll learn to lie or hide who you are. Don't be afraid to end
a relationship if you have doubts.
—Eleanor

One of the first things that you can do during your engagement to prepare for sex is to start talking about sex with your fiancé. I know this sounds counterintuitive, because now that you're closer to the wedding day, it will be harder than ever to remain chaste, and sitting down for long talks about sex with the man you love doesn't seem like the key to abstinence. Well, I haven't told you what you should be talking about. With the help of a premarital counselor or mature Christian friend, it's time to discuss the difficult topics of past sexual sin, STIs, and porn.

Premarital Counseling A must

There's one thing that I find incredibly surprising and fascinating about all the stories I hear from women about their honeymoons: of the couples who have the most "successful" first six months of married sex, almost all participated in premarital counseling that involved detailed teaching about sex.

The more you can inform and prepare yourself for sex, the better. The best possible way to do this seems to be with your fiancé in the company of a professional counselor or an older, wiser Christian who has good information about sex and is not afraid to tell you everything you need to know. So ask around until you find a counselor with this kind of premarital training, and spend the money or take the time to make this a priority during your engagement.

Past Sexual Activity ~~Rough~~

Even if you and your fiancé have not had sex with each other, one or the other of you may still have had past sexual activity. Your fiancé deserves to know your sexual past and you deserve to know his. Marriage is about intimacy, and without openness and vulnerability, even about past sin, this will not be possible. It's especially important to come clean if you have had any kind of sex with another person (vaginal, oral, manual, or anal intercourse), if you have a history of masturbation or pornography, if you had been sexually abused, or if you have struggled with same-sex attraction.

As you navigate these potentially treacherous waters, remember the beautiful truth that the Lord exchanges our ashes for something beautiful! His name is Redeemer, and that's not without reason. He can redeem anything, even our sexual sin, and turn it into something that glorifies himself (see Isa. 61:3). If either you or your fiancé is not a virgin, remember that because of Jesus's blood you are declared righteous before God.

While those with past sexual activity may struggle with guilt, virgins may face a different kind of struggle. Sometimes virgins believe that because of their years of abstinence and perseverance, they deserve to be married to a virgin, and may discover feelings of resentment or bitterness toward their non-virgin fiancé. Instead, remember that none of us are righteous for any reason other than the blood of Jesus. We depend on Jesus, not our own good actions, for our "goodness." If we begin to feel pride in our righteousness, that righteousness becomes a liability.

In either case, frank discussions with a premarital counselor will be helpful in communicating about past sexual sin and processing your thoughts and feelings as you do so.

When we realized we were serious about each other, my boyfriend came to me one evening, tear-stained, and took me on a walk. He explained how he wasn't a Christian until he was eighteen and was sexually active before. He told me he would give me as long as I needed to think it through. And that he was okay with me breaking off the relationship if I couldn't be with him because of it. And he gave me the name of a girl he knew who I could talk with about it, because her fiancé wasn't a virgin either.

I talked with the girl, prayed and processed deeply through it all. I kept thinking, "That was what he used to be. That isn't him now." I cried. I felt so, so, so sad. I felt like I would be compared to their bodies. I felt naive as he would know how to do it, and I wouldn't.

He called me a few days later, broken, and told me that when we spoke earlier it seemed that I hadn't really realized the full extent. I had thought it was just one or two girls, but it was more than that. I'm amazed now that he had to put himself out there again to make sure I knew the reality beforehand. He has always been so honest about sex, about himself.

Amazing

But it felt simple to me. I decided that what God had done for me, I would do for him. That it was foundational to our marriage. And I haven't brought it up against him ever, not during sex, not during arguments. We have talked about it openly, and he says that because I never treated him any differently in any way, that he even feels like that was someone else.

I share the times when I feel sad about it, and we walk through the feelings together. It helps to never ask details, to never ask names, to not know. It is so powerful for us, so intimate in a crazy way. It's not part of our sex life anymore . . . we've walked through the doors and felt this crazy grace for each other. And I would add that I think that the pride or anger or sin issues that I have in my life are as destructive to our marriage as his past sexual sins, because mine are still active. That makes them possibly even more destructive.

To make this realization has been a big part of the journey: who we are to each other as husband and wife heals or hurts far more than who we used to be before we were together. And anyway, I'M THE WOMAN who knows my man's body . . . those girls just got him as a high school guy. I know him NOW, for the man he is. And we get oneness like they never knew.
— Andi

Before I knew Jesus, I was a very sexually immoral person. Sadly, I lost my virginity at age fourteen and slept with many people, men and women, until age nineteen, when I died with Jesus in baptism. I even contracted a few STIs, which thankfully were curable. When my husband and I became engaged, I confessed all these things to him. Praise God, my husband has the mind of Christ and knows that I am a totally new creation in Jesus, that the old person I once was, is dead forever.

My past really has not affected our marriage to a great degree. I gave myself away so much before I knew Jesus, but to be quite honest, the Lord has restored it and redeemed that more than I can explain to another human being.

The only thing that was bothersome was that before I got married, I knew how to have sex. On our honeymoon I wanted everything to be new for the both of us. I didn't want to take the lead because I had previous experience (although it had been 10 whole years since I had sex. Praise God!).

I know that Christ has forgiven me completely and has healed me from the emotional damage of having sex with people. I am righteous before God; therefore, I know that I am righteous before my husband as well. I have felt as though the Lord has brought great and deep cleansing to my heart through having sex with my husband.
—Eliza

Sexually Transmitted Infections

If you're dealing with past sexual sin in your relationship, another difficult subject you need to discuss is STIs (sexually transmitted infections) and STDs (sexually transmitted diseases). The scary truth is that a man or a woman can have an STI without any visible symptoms. That means that even if you had sex years ago and don't feel like anything is wrong with your body, you could still have an STI. For your own health and the health of the man you love, get tested for STIs.

If your fiancé is the one who isn't a virgin, ask him to get tested for STIs. Some men may be very uncomfortable with this, especially if they have no visible signs of an STI, but frankly, this is a hill to die on. STIs are serious stuff, causing pain, discomfort, and potentially destroying a woman's ability to have children. If that's your future, you'll want to walk into it with your eyes open.

Pornography Usage

Recent studies report that a chilling 15 percent of Christian women and 64 percent of Christian men are watching porn at least once a month.[15] Because pornography usage is so widespread, porn's distorted views of sex have deeply impacted the sexuality of men and woman. "Porn teaches [a man] that sex should be accessible at any time, a woman is to be dominated and used, the goal of sex is for him to orgasm, [and] when he is no longer fulfilled, he should find someone/something new that excites him."[16]

Porn teaches a woman that "if you want a relationship, you must give him whatever kind of sex he wants, your self-worth is tied to your appearance and sexual performance, a man could never be fully committed to you mentally or physically, [and] that verbal and physical abuse is normal and permissible in relationships."[17]

Since nearly every person is either directly or indirectly affected by porn, it should be a topic of discussion during engagement. Confess any pornography usage and discuss the ways that porn has directly or indirectly affected you. If either you or your fiancé use porn on a regular basis (once a month or more), consider calling off the wedding so that the one struggling can get help. Pornography is incredibly damaging to the sexuality of the person using it, not to mention that person's married partner, and the kindest thing you can do for yourself or your fiancé is to get the help needed to overcome this addiction.

Non-Negotiables

As you and your fiancé communicate about past sexual sin, STIs, and pornography, you may see some red flags about each other or your relationship. While there are a host of issues to discuss regarding your marriage at large, here we'll discuss a few sexual issues that may be non-negotiables for someone entering into marriage with another person.

Discuss your expectations about children. Do you want to have them? How many do you expect to have? Do you want to adopt? If you encounter infertility issues, what medical steps will you take to overcome these issues?

Are either of you addicted to sex, pornography, or masturbation? If so, this will have far-reaching effects on your relationship and you should consider whether a marriage is appropriate. Instead, give the person struggling with addiction the freedom, time, and support to seek help. It is possible to change, but it takes a lot of time, help, and work.

Ask each other about your expectations about sex in marriage. What do you believe it means to be chaste in marriage? How often do you expect to have sex? What kind of sexual activity do you look forward to? What sexual activity are you uncomfortable with? What sexual activity do you believe to be sinful in marriage?

State your beliefs about consent to each other. Will you both respect each other's "no" concerning sexual activity? Have either of you pushed for or forced sexual activity on the other when he or she was unwilling? Do you commit to only pursing sexual activity if you have both communicated a willingness and openness to it? Will you stop any sexual activity at any time if the other expresses "no"?

The answers to these questions are extremely important—a disagreement may signify that marriage is not a good option for you as a couple. It is possible to love someone very much and yet it not be right to marry him. Marriage is for two people who choose to come together in a covenant, before God, to love and respect each other for their whole lives, in order to glorify God. Seriously consider any red flags you encounter during premarital counseling, knowing that not only your life but also the glory of God is at stake.

Preparation

Think of it this way: You'd never consider entering a marathon without training beforehand, would you? You wouldn't expect to ride a bike for a hundred miles if you had never ridden a bike before.
                                                    —Dr. Kevin Leman

As your wedding day nears, you can begin to turn your attention to the actual act of sex. Here you'll find some simple, practical advice for preparing both your body and your mind for the act of love that you and your fiancé will soon share.

Pregnancy Awareness

Don't forget that whenever you have sex, there is the potential to create life, a brand-new soul that will exist for eternity. Remember to pray and seek God's leading with your fiancé about the possibility of starting a family.

Because there's always a potential for pregnancy when sexually active, you will need to have it on your radar. Refrain from smoking (which creates an increased risk of miscarriage), binge drinking, and taking some medications (for acne, cholesterol, depression, or high blood pressure) that can result in birth defects.

Together, prayerfully and carefully consider if you want to use birth control. If you do, there are a number of options, and Dr. Fogarty has kindly broken down the most popular ones for us:

1. Condoms

A condom is a thin (usually latex) sleeve put over the erect penis to catch semen so that it does not enter the vagina. This is referred to as a barrier method of birth control. Condoms are easy to use and easily available. However, they do not protect from STIs and are not 100 percent effective at preventing pregnancy even in lab tests. Studies show that with typical use, they are 86 percent effective at preventing pregnancy during the first year of usage.[18]

2. The Pill

Various forms of birth control fall under this category, but the basic idea is that you take hormones that simulate a pregnancy within your own body. This prevents your body from ovulating, thus making it impossible to get pregnant. Make sure to choose a form that can't be used as an abortifacient. Some people can't use the pill because the hormones make them feel sick or overly emotional, but most people can handle a low-dose birth control pill.

3. Fertility Awareness Method

By observing and charting your body's signals, you determine the exact date of ovulation each month and then either abstain or use contraceptives (such as condoms) during your days of fertility each month. This method depends upon self-control and organization, so there is a huge margin for error. However, if you have a regular cycle and you're both committed to planning and talking it out, FAM can be a great way to prevent or plan a pregnancy.

4. *Intrauterine Device (IUD)*

An IUD is a device (often T-shaped) inserted into the uterus, which works by making the environment fatal to sperm. In some cases, the IUD also affects the lining of the uterus, preventing implantation.This is a long-term birth control option, and usually only recommended if you don't want children for several years. It has a high success rate and a high satisfaction rating with users, but because of some rare yet severe side effects, be sure to fully research this option before deciding if it's right for you.

5. *Morning-After Pill*

This is a pill taken after having sex that will terminate a pregnancy within three to five days after conception. As Dr. Fogarty says, this is, "Too sorry, too late." Please do not choose to end a pregnancy, no matter how strongly you feel about waiting to have children. You can trust God, knowing that he is powerful and good, to guide you through parenthood.

There are many other forms of birth control as well, and it's a good idea to research on your own until you find the method that's best for you and your future husband. Talk to a doctor and other wise and godly couples who can tell you their own opinions on the matter. Make sure to talk this out together and come to a decision that you're both confident about.

Doctor's Visit

Schedule an appointment with your OB/GYN about three to six months before your wedding.

Your doctor may ask about your plans for birth control. If you're planning to get pregnant, you'll need to tell her so that she can be prepared and can tell you if there's anything you need to know. If you want her help finding a good birth control option, here's your chance.

Ask her any questions you may have and then decide what you'd like to do (or go home to think about it). She can write you a prescription for birth control that you can take to a pharmacy to get filled.

You may wish to ask your doctor for an antibiotic to have on hand during your honeymoon week. Lots of women get urinary tract infections when they start having sex for the first time. Most women don't have access to a doctor during their honeymoons, so it's a good idea to be prepared. Almost any gynecologist will be happy to keep you healthy in this way.

Along with these two things, have your normal exam to make sure your body is healthy.

Stretching

Your vagina will likely need stretching in order to accommodate your husband's penis. Since every woman's size and shape is different, some women will require more stretching than others. Determine how much stretching you'll need and what method you'll use to stretch yourself. There are two ways you can do this:

The first way is to stretch your vagina with your husband's help. This means waiting for your wedding night to let him use his penis (or fingers) to gently stretch your vagina.

Be prepared for it to take anywhere from one to four days before you are able to achieve coitus, or vaginal intercourse. If you've previously been able to use tampons, it might only take a couple tries. If you can't use tampons, this probably means that your hymen is thick and covers a good portion of your vaginal opening. In this case, it will take much longer (think in terms of days or even weeks) before you can have vaginal sex. Be sure to go very slowly. Think of it as stretching instead of "sexing." Pushing through the hymen will tear it instead of stretching it, and you will probably bleed and experience a lot of pain.

I only recommend this method if you and your fiancé have agreed upon this method with the full understanding that you will not have sex the first time you try. Only use this method if you're both committed to stretching out your hymen patiently and slowly so that you do not injure yourself when trying to have sex. (Remember, tearing your hymen is an injury, not the act of losing your virginity. Having sex can stretch your hymen to the point of discomfort, but it should never be painful.)

The second way is to stretch yourself out in the weeks leading up to your wedding. Dr. Fogarty has a couple great exercises for this.

If you have never been able to use a tampon, buy a multi-size box of tampons. Draw a warm bath, then insert half of a junior-sized tampon into your vagina, and get into the water. The water will cause the tampon to expand, gradually stretching your vagina. Over the course of several "bath sessions," go from junior size to regular, then from regular to super, and finally from super to super-plus. This will enable you to use a tampon on a regular basis.

If you are able to use a tampon (or have completed the "bath sessions"), use your fingers to continue stretching your vagina. Slowly and gently insert one finger into your vagina. Once you are able to insert one finger easily, then insert two and gradually work up to three fingers. The stretching feels a little like a burning sensation, but it doesn't hurt. Be gentle with yourself as you gradually work up to three fingers.

I recommend stretching yourself out in the days leading up to your wedding night. This will prepare your vagina for sex and will insure that you will experience less pain. Using your finger to stretch your hymen does not affect your virginity. It's preparing your body for sex in the same way that you would exercise, primp, and clean yourself in preparation. If you stretch your vagina, there is a better chance you will be able to have sex on your wedding night with minimal pain, which will be more pleasurable for both you and your new husband.

Your Period

Try to calculate whether you'll be on your period at any time during your honeymoon. If you think there's a possibility that you will start bleeding, there are a couple things you can do.

If you're taking an oral contraceptive, talk to your doctor about using it to skip a period. Some women's bodies reject this, which is why I advise talking to your doctor, but the idea is that instead of taking the week of placebo pills, you start your next pack, thereby "skipping" your period and continuing on to your next cycle.

Talk to your fiancé about the possibility of being on your period. Discuss whether you'll try to have vaginal intercourse or if you'll use other forms of sex during this time. Dr. Fogarty advises against sex during your period, "because your cervix opens up wider and it increases the risk of vaginal infections. You can get infection up in your uterus." If you can't resist, be sure to clean up properly before and after sex.

There are lots of creative and incredible ways to make love with your husband besides vaginal intercourse. So don't worry if you're bleeding too heavily to have sex this way during those first few days. You will find plenty of ways to be intimate and pleasure each other. (Part Three is loaded with ideas!) Besides, you now have a lifetime of sex together, so there's no rush. Relax into the uniqueness of your own experience.

Flipping the Switch *So true*

> A lot of the difficulty that we had in the first six months was just me trying to adjust to this new life. I was so naive and such a rule follower that I had to totally reprogram my mind that sex was okay.
>
> —Katie

In my interviews, I heard many women refer to engagement as a time when they struggled with "flipping the switch." They use this term because it begins to dawn on them that after years of suppressing their sex drive and viewing sex as a bad thing, one night it will be suddenly, irrevocably good. Not only good, but encouraged.

It's easy after all those years of ignoring your sexual feelings to feel like you don't even have them anymore. You may have learned to relate to your fiancé in a completely non-sexual way. Or perhaps it's hard to think of sex as anything but bad. Here are a couple reminders for you that might help:

You Will Not "Lose" Your Virginity

Like we discussed in Part One, don't consider yourself a virgin who is about to lose something. Don't even think of yourself as being pure "until" your wedding night. If married sex is godly, then it's no different than being an unmarried virgin. You are going from one good thing to another.

You are soon to partake in one of God's greatest gifts. Because of Jesus' death for your sins, you have a pure heart and body as a single woman, so you will have a pure heart and body after you're married. Purity has nothing to do with whether or not you've had sex, but whether or not you're someone who participates in sex the way God intended.

Let Yourself Look Forward to Sex

One afternoon when I was engaged, I was taking a nap and was suddenly deeply aroused and filled with anticipation for the moment when I could have sex with my fiancé. It was hard to know how to process and deal with these emotions and feelings. I got out of bed, opened my journal, and wrote in giant letters, "I WANT TO HAVE SEX." Then, I basically said/shouted the same thing to God in a prayer.

It helped to acknowledge that what I wanted wasn't bad, to process my feelings, and to know that God would help lead me through the difficult waiting period until the time when he had ordained for us to be together (after we were married).

Communicating with your fiancé about past and future sexual activity, preparing for sex with your husband, and finding healthy ways to "flip the switch" are all ways to be a darling while you're engaged. As you center yourself in God's great love for you, believing that his ways are the best ways, you can find the desire and the strength to be chaste during your engagement.

6

The Honeymoon

*Our honeymoon will shine our life long: its beams will only
fade over your grave or mine.*
—Charlotte Brontë

. . . and they shall become one flesh.
—Genesis 2:24 ESV

On your honeymoon, you find yourself at the edge of a whole new sexual lifestyle. You and your new husband have just bound yourselves to each other in a covenant and made a promise to be each other's companion for the rest of your lives. Of that moment, the book of Malachi says, "Did he not make them one, with a portion of the Spirit in their union?" (Mal. 2:15 ESV). Your marriage is a sacred thing, with the very Spirit of God hovering over you. And now, in this place, you unite even your physical body with that of your husband.

Forget your past, if you've had sex with someone else before, if he's had sex with someone else before, if you've had sex with each other. Now, in this moment, you partake in sex as God intended—the unification of a man and a woman, in the context of marriage, for the glory of God.

Planning Your Honeymoon

*Sexually speaking, there are few worse ways to start a
marriage than with a wedding.*
　　　　　　　—Dr. Kevin Leman

Planning your honeymoon will be fun to talk and dream about with your
fiancé. While you may need to discuss travel dates, locations, and hotel
reservations early on in your engagement, I'd highly recommend
waiting to ask the more intimate questions (especially specific desires
for the honeymoon night) until a few weeks prior to the wedding. It will
only cause you torment if you have to wait too long for the fulfillment
of your desires.

Once you're within two to four weeks of your honeymoon night,
have a few conversations with each other in which you address these
questions (perhaps in the presence of a premarital counselor or trusted
friend):

- What are your expectations for the honeymoon night? What are
  your hopes? Fears?
- Are you looking forward to your honeymoon night or do you feel
  nervous or scared?
- Do you expect to spend a lot of time at your wedding reception
  celebrating with family and friends? Would you rather hurry
  away from the crowd?
- Once you are alone after your wedding, do you want to have sex
  immediately? Would you rather eat, shower, or relax together
  first? What kind of foreplay would you like?
- Is there anything you'd like on hand to make the experience more
  romantic? Music? Candles? Champagne? Perhaps spend some
  time telling each other what you love about each other? Read
  Song of Solomon together?

- Will you wear your wedding dress the first time you have sex? Or will you wear lingerie? Or will you be naked? What about your fiancé? Should he be naked? Should he have nice boxers? Do you want to undress each other?

If you haven't already, discuss your opinions and beliefs about sexual activity. Spend some time getting informed about different kinds of sex, different positions, and different factors and ideas that help a man and woman have pleasurable sex. (Part Three of this book contains plenty on these topics). Then talk to each other about what you both are learning and how it's shaping your thinking about sex. Share what you are looking forward to trying, what you may need some time before trying, and what you would never like to try.

Try to answer all these questions as honestly and openly as you can, and not just tell him what you think he wants to hear. Truly listen to your fiancé's answers. Come to decisions together.

It can feel scary if you find that the two of you don't agree about something, especially something as sensitive as sex. But instead of becoming fearful or taking it personally, see the conflict as an opportunity to become more intimate through the process of good communication, selfless giving, and honesty. If you take the time to creatively find a solution to your conflict, you will likely become more bonded than ever, even if the disagreement was difficult at the time!

Looking Your Best

*They may talk of a comet, or a burning mountain, or some such
bagatelle; but to me a modest woman, dressed out in all her
finery, is the most tremendous object of the whole creation.*
—Oliver Goldsmith

If you read Part One of this book, then you already know how to care for your body, so make sure to schedule time in the days leading up to your wedding to relax and ready your body for your lover.

The week of my wedding, my grandmother gave me a gift card for a manicure, and it was such a blessing to be able to leave the chaos of wedding preparations to spend an hour in silence as someone massaged and pampered my hands. My nails were shiny and perfect on our wedding day.

Also, after our rehearsal dinner, everyone started playing games and talking, but I snuck away and went to my parents' house. I spent over an hour scrubbing myself clean, moisturizing, shaving, and tweezing until I was soft and smooth all over. I slipped into bed before anyone even came home and got a good eight hours of sleep before our wedding day. It was so peaceful, exactly what I needed to ready both my body and my mind.

However, this was what made me feel beautiful and ready for my husband. Maybe for you, it would be way more exciting to get a special tattoo, for your husband's eyes only. Or perhaps you want to spend time sewing a piece of lingerie for the first night. Find something that fits you, that makes you feel beautiful, and that you know will excite your new husband.

Think of your body as a gift that you're giving to the one you love more than anyone else in the world on one of the most important days of your relationship. As hardly any woman is completely satisfied with her body, this idea has the potential to make you feel nervous or pressured. But the truth is that he will be thrilled with your body, however he finds it.

And as you ready your body for your wedding day, don't do it for all the people who will be watching you walk down the aisle; do it for the man who loves you so much he wants to marry you. Take pride in the body God gave you! Watch your husband get drunk with love for you. Find satisfaction in the joy that you are giving him with your body. Do it out of love, not out of a need for praise or because you feel pressure or out of a desire for power over him. Do it out of love, always and only.

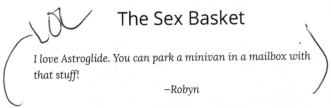

The Sex Basket

I love Astroglide. You can park a minivan in a mailbox with that stuff!

—Robyn

There is a certain amount of "gear" that goes along with sex, especially those first few days or weeks. Find yourself a basket or box and fill it with all the things you'll want handy. This will be an easy and discreet way of toting the items with you wherever you go. Also, once you get to your new home, you can put the basket by the side of your bed—one very useful decoration!

Sexy Stuff

Setting the mood is an important part of sex and can help jump-start your sex drive. Lingerie, champagne or sparkling juice, music, candles, and flowers can all create an environment that turns you on.

Antibiotics

As mentioned, you may want to bring along an antibiotic. Some doctors recommend popping one on your wedding night and maybe the next two or three days as well. This will wipe out any infection before it starts. (However, remember that taking antibiotics affects some birth control medicine, so don't take an antibiotic if you're relying on an oral contraceptive to prevent pregnancy.)

Lubricant

The best forms of lubrication are all-natural oils like olive oil, vegetable oil, and coconut oil. They're gentle on sensitive skin, they allow sperm to get through, and cut down on the number of infections. Also, coconut oil can fight yeast infections (not to mention it smells and tastes great). There are also many kinds of synthetic lubricants you can buy at the store. I recommend a water-based lubricant, as they tend to be less sticky.

There are some lubricants that advertise other benefits. For example, they may say that they increase pleasure by creating a "warming sensation." But Dr. Fogarty says, "I've had patients come in with terrible chemical burns because of allergic reactions to these lubricants. Even if you don't have a reaction, make sure you wash it off afterwards. Otherwise, if you have sensitive skin, you could break out or get a bladder infection."

Cranberry Juice

Bring along a bottle of cranberry juice and sip it throughout the days of your honeymoon. The acid in the cranberries will help maintain the proper pH balance in your vagina and prevent infections.

Towels

Sex can get messy. I'll explain more later, but you may wish to have towels on hand to clean up with. Some people spread a large towel, blanket, or sheet on top of the bed before sex. Most people use some combination of tissues, toilet paper, flushable wet wipes, or a hand towel.

Birth Control

Don't forget to bring your birth control. If you're on the pill, don't forget your pills. If you're using condoms, don't forget your condoms. If you're using the fertility awareness method, don't forget your thermometer and charts.

No matter what your method, go ahead and throw in a couple condoms no matter what, in case you forget to take your medicine one day, or if you're not sure if you're fertile. Having condoms available is convenient if you have an accident with another method of birth control.

The First Time

It's such a fun, scary, exciting, a little embarrassing, great thing to finally be naked with the man of your dreams on the wedding night!
—Clara

During the marriage ceremony, you form a covenant with your new husband. Biblically speaking, a covenant is different from a promise or contract, which is between two parties, because a covenant is made between three parties—you, your husband, and God. Jesus states that at this moment, God bonds the two of you into one, spiritually uniting your souls (see Matt. 19:4–6). Sometime after the wedding, in the most private and personal ceremony of all, you consummate this bond in a physical way when you have sex for the first time.

What to Remember

There are an infinite number of ways that your wedding night might take place, and you won't be able to predict what will happen. Appendix A contains over a dozen honeymoon stories from Christian women that will hopefully give you a better idea of the variety of ways that sex plays out for a loving couple. However, there are a few things that are true for almost every couple having sex for the first time.

1. Sex Won't Last Very Long

Your husband has waited a long time for this night, and just the sight of your beautiful, naked body may make him orgasm. (Once a man orgasms, it will take anywhere from several minutes to hours before he can have sex again.) He may be able to last longer, but the touch of you, the sight of you, the smell of you will make it overwhelmingly wonderful for him, and he may climax very quickly. Be prepared for this. Please don't judge him. Drink up and enjoy the moments, and know that there are so many more ahead of you.

2. Your Own Pleasure Is Important

Too often, it's assumed that having sex is two people coming together until the man orgasms. But this isn't true. The Lord designed sex to be between two people for the purpose of intimacy and service and pleasure. It's important for your husband and for you to remember that your own experience during sex is important. If your husband orgasms quickly, this doesn't mean that sex is over. Your own pleasure and climax, as well as your husband's, should be the goal. Don't be afraid to expect and ask for this. It's not selfish, it's part of God's design.

3. Intimacy, Not Sex, Is Your Goal

Even during the sexual act there can be broken expectations, dashed hopes, and hurt feelings. But no matter how your honeymoon goes, you can still experience successful sex if you choose to be intimate and vulnerable with each other.

Here's what I mean. Let's say you arrive at your hotel after the wedding, exhausted and high-strung, feeling sweaty instead of sexy, and you're just not in the mood. What do you do? You could suppress your feelings and pretend you don't have them, forcing it so that he can have sex and you don't "ruin the evening." Or you could hold him at arm's length, close yourself off to him until he gets the hint and you both go to bed.

But instead, what if you saw your mixed emotions as a chance for further intimacy? Let him know how you feel. Invite him into your head and your heart, and see if together you can come up with a good solution for the evening. Maybe you cuddle or shower together instead, getting used to each other's bodies. Maybe you settle down beside each other and drink a glass of wine. (Who knows? You may suddenly feel relaxed and turned on, and then decide to go for it!)

But at the end of that, wouldn't you feel like it was perfect? Even though you had started out feeling far from intimate or sexy, your step toward intimacy (by communicating with him) led you both toward intimacy, regardless of whether or not you had sex.

What to Do

Before your honeymoon, I suggest reading Part Three of this book, which will educate you on what happens during sex, how to become sexually aroused, what gives women and men pleasure during sex, and some common pitfalls. Once you do this, you'll be prepared to have a great sex life with your husband, but here are a few specific suggestions for that first time you come together:

1. Don't Arrive Exhausted

Reserve quality time, before you're too exhausted, to fully engage in the consummation of your marriage. If you arrive at your hotel at 11:30 p.m. after a night of conversation and dancing, you won't be firing on all cylinders. It might be difficult to fully engage sexually or you may become overly emotional purely because you're too tired. Perhaps plan an afternoon or early evening wedding.

2. Don't Plan Long Travel on Your Wedding Day

If you do have to fly or drive to your honeymoon, see that it's either a short trip or that it happens the next day. Again, don't arrive at your honeymoon suite exhausted and emotionally spent. Save something for the beautiful act of intimacy and marriage that you're about to partake in.

3. Give Yourself Time and Privacy

Once locked up in your room, you don't want to be bothered or interrupted for the foreseeable future. Whether you're in a hotel, a house, a bed-and-breakfast, or a tent, make sure you'll have privacy for a very long time. If you ever become concerned that someone might bang on the door or hear you, or if you have some kind of time constraint, it can make you feel tense, which will easily kill the mood.

4. Go Slowly

Don't rush the experience of making love; instead, reserve lots of time for communication and foreplay. But more than anything, go slowly when you begin vaginal intercourse. If done too quickly, you could experience pain or even injure your hymen. Clearly communicate to each other as you attempt intercourse for the first time, using phrases like, "Go slowly," "Stop," "May I...?" "A little more," etc.

On Hollywood

Real sex isn't quite as smooth as in the movies—but that makes it better.

—Brooke

There's one thing that you should know—your sex will not look like the movies. Hollywood lies about sex. I'm not trying to say that Hollywood has different opinions about sex than I do (although that is true). I'm saying that Hollywood lies on screen about what they know to be true in real life.

For example, what's the most typical way for Hollywood to communicate that two people have had sex with each other? Waking up naked in bed together the next morning, right? So apparently they had sex, then rolled over and fell asleep, letting all that sticky mess dry on them overnight. Just thinking about it makes me feel kind of queasy. Plus, that means they would probably all have raging bladder infections! But it's not romantic to show a couple having sex and then promptly stuffing tissue in their crotches and hopping to the bathroom. So even though almost all couples (including Hollywood stars) clean up after sex, movies don't show it.

Also, Hollywood rarely shows a couple stopping to put on a condom. Hollywood shows couples rolling around under the sheets together, even though this is nearly impossible to pull off during coitus. Hollywood doesn't show any awkward sex positions, even though these are often the most pleasurable and widely used.

Partly, they're not to blame. There are many realities of life that don't appear on the big screen, simply because it doesn't make a good story. We don't need to see a couple doing laundry to know that everyone must wash their clothes. We don't need to see someone stewing over their W-2s to know that everyone must pay their taxes.

In the same way, movies and TV rarely show what sex actually looks like, because like all of life, sex is messy and complex when it's between real people. But in that messy complexity, you'll find the warm embrace of a real man and the ultimate joy of true love.

Part Three

Married Darlings

7

The Basics of Sex

Sex isn't just improv and impulse. It's more like a dance, and certain steps are just better than others.
    —Georgia

How aroused I am before intercourse usually affects how big my orgasm will be.
    —Anna

In Part One, we discovered that sex was designed in the Garden of Eden to be between two people, a man and a woman, within the context of a covenantal marriage, and that it is very good. The purpose behind this unique design is to strengthen and ratify the covenant, to create unity between two separate people, to create new life, and to give pleasure. Ultimately, this good gift was given to us as a picture of Jesus and the church, a way to catch a glimpse of the self-giving, faithful love of our God, so that we might glorify and enjoy him.

Embracing God's will for sex is a way of opening yourself up to the best sex. If it seems limiting or suppressing, it should be seen as limiting a superficial experience and only suppressing self-absorption and self-destructive behavior. For as Lauren F. Winner says, "Life lived inside the contours of God's law humanizes us and makes us beautiful. It makes us creatures living well in the created order. It gives us the opportunity to become who we are meant to be."[19]

What Makes Great Sex?

It might sound shocking, but it's true: God doesn't turn his eyes when a married couple goes to bed. It only stands to reason that we shouldn't turn our eyes from God when we share intimate moments with our spouse.
—Gary Thomas

Once you are married, you get the delight of discovering sex with your husband. You can excitedly and anxiously begin the work of creating a beautiful sex life with your husband. But what, exactly, does that mean? What makes great sex?

I can't help but think of a scene from a movie, two passionate lovers clasped in each other's arms, lusty and blinded by the thrill of the forbidden. In this scene, "great sex" means excitement, passion, butterflies in your stomach, even risk.

To be honest, these are all things that are hard to come by in marriage. By its very nature, marriage has taken away both the threat of risk and the thrill of first-time experiences. Has our decision to wait to have sex until marriage robbed us of the best sex by stealing forever the potential for excitement, passion, and risk? Is that what it means to have great sex? What did God have in mind?

In their wonderful book on marriage, Tim and Kathy Keller write,

> One of the reasons we believe in our culture that sex should always and only be the result of great passion is that so many people today have learned how to have sex outside of marriage, and this is a very different experience than having sex inside it. Outside of marriage, sex is accompanied by a desire to impress or entice someone. It is something like the thrill of the hunt. When you are seeking to draw in someone you don't

So important [handwritten marginalia]

know, it injects risk, uncertainty, and pressure to the lovemaking that quickens the heartbeat and stirs the emotions. If "great sex" is defined in this way, then marriage— the "piece of paper"—will indeed stifle that particular kind of thrill. But this defines sexual sizzle in terms that would be impossible to maintain in any case. The fact is that "the thrill of the hunt" is not the only kind of thrill or passion available, nor is it the best.

[My wife] Kathy and I were virgins when we married. Even in our day, that may have been the minority experience, but that meant that on our wedding night we were not in any position to try to impress or entice one another. All we were trying to do was to tenderly express with our bodies the oneness we had first begun feeling as friends and which had then grown stronger and deeper as we fell in love. Frankly, that night I was clumsy and awkward and fell asleep anxious and discouraged. Sex was frustrating at first. It was the frustration of an artist who has in his head a picture or a story but lacks the skills to express it.

However, we had fortunately not learned to use sex to impress, nor to mix the thrill of the dangerous and the forbidden with sexual stimulation and mistake it for love. With sex, we were trying to be vulnerable to each other, to give each other the gift of bare-faced rejoicing in one another, and to know the pleasure of giving one another pleasure. And as the weeks went by, and then the years, we did it better and better. Yes, it means making love sometimes when one or even both of you are not "in the mood." But sex in a marriage, done to give joy rather than to impress, can change your mood on the spot. The best sex makes you want to weep tears of joy, not bask in the glow of a good performance.[20]

While passion is surely a beautiful and rewarding aspect of sex, could it be that God's plan all along was something different and more wonderful? His plan intends sex to be the means to an end, a way to give and receive the sacrificial and infinite love of Christ for the church. Instead of passion, make intimacy the plumb line in your sex life.

And as you approach every pleasant encounter and every heartbreaking conflict within your sex life as a way to love and bond with your husband, you will glimpse a picture of God himself. When you make yourself vulnerable to your husband, taking off every barrier of defense, even your very clothes, with no guarantee that he will respond perfectly to you, then you enact the vulnerable love of God that reveals itself with no guarantee of our reciprocity. When you choose to accept and love your husband, no matter how many angry outbursts, how big his belly, how high his hairline, how apathetic his romance, you participate in the unconditional love of Jesus, who forgives you a debt of a hundred billion dollars. When you choose to serve your husband, to give him pleasure and joy regardless of whether or not you'll get a compliment or a back rub or an orgasm in return, you will discover the heart of Jesus, who went so far as to endure physical torment in order to bring us peace and healing (see Isa. 53:5).

But now imagine two such people exhibiting the vulnerability, acceptance, and selfless service of Christ, simultaneously, for as long as they both shall live. Think of the pleasure, the gratitude, the blessing that this would bring. You see now why Keller says that this kind of sex ends in tears of joy. Profound intimacy can be found in sex when we participate in it in the way that God intended.

Let intimacy be the path you choose for your sex life. Let sex deepen and grow the relationship that you have with your husband, the man you love who has given himself to you. And may your journey lead you straight to the heart of God.

The Human Sexual Response Cycle

Our premarital counselor drew us a picture of the Human
Sexual Response Cycle and explained it to us. It has been the
biggest help for us; I am able to orgasm almost every time we
have sex. Incredible.

—Nina

Whenever a man or woman has sex, his or her mind, heart, and body goes through something called the Human Sexual Response Cycle.[21] It is what happens from the moment when your new husband gets sight of you in your lacy lingerie for the very first time to the moment that you both get off the bed and head to the bathroom to clean up afterward. I'll break it down:

The Excitement Phase

There are so many things that can trigger the excitement phase. Sometimes it's a particularly pleasant kiss. Sometimes your husband sees your body and it starts. Sometimes your husband says something sweet to you and then later, when he hugs you, it begins. Whatever the trigger is, it causes huge reactions in your body.

For you, it can feel like many different things. Perhaps you suddenly feel wet in your vagina, which is your body secreting lubrication to prepare the channel for sex. Maybe you have heightened feeling in your genital area (your clitoris is swelling, your vagina is expanding, and your outer labia flattens and opens to reveal the vaginal opening). Your nipples may pop up and show through your bra. Your skin may flush. Suddenly, you realize, you'd like to have sex.

For a man, it's more obvious. His penis becomes erect; he'd like to have sex.

It's important for you both to go through the excitement phase before moving on. If you don't have your own excitement phase (if, for example, he initiates intimacy) before you move on, then it will be

[handwritten: easy for guys in any situation]

incredibly hard for you to have an orgasm. Use lots of foreplay and happy, sexy thoughts to produce your own excitement phase.

The Plateau Phase *[handwritten: Sometimes difficult]*

Once you're both aroused, you continue to the plateau phase. This is what most people think of when they think of "sex." It's basically anything that happens between arousal and orgasm. After you become aroused, you begin to have sex in order to build tension. This sexual tension will build and build until you have an orgasm.

In A Celebration of Sex, Douglas Rosenau makes a helpful suggestion: "Research has found that a man, if actively thrusting, will often climax in less than two minutes while a woman will take much longer to reach an orgasm. The wise couple intersperses intercourse throughout the plateau phase as the husband starts and stops and keeps his arousal on a plateau without peaking too soon. Both husband and wife can learn to approach an orgasm and then back off as they maintain the plateau phase for extended periods of pleasurable and sensuous lovemaking."[22]

This phase can feel like a series of hills and valleys or even waves. Your sexual tension and feeling of pleasure builds up and then will suddenly be gone. Keep going and the tension will build again, each time with greater intensity.

Now, because of the location of the clitoris, two-thirds of women cannot reach the orgasm phase by intercourse.[23] That means that you'll reach the orgasm phase through your husband's manual or oral stimulation (more on that in Chapter 9).

The Orgasm Phase

The plateau phase will eventually build up so much tension that there will be an involuntary release in the orgasm phase. Once this occurs, just relax, forget yourself, and enjoy every last sensation.

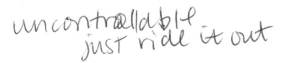

uncontrollable — just ride it out

It's nearly impossible to describe an orgasm, so sometimes women wonder whether or not they've had an orgasm. This probably means they haven't. You'll know it when you have one. Think of it like a Fourth of July fireworks show. The lights are dazzling and beautiful, and when they're especially stunning, you think, "Was that the finale?" But they keep coming and bursting with even greater brightness, and you wonder, "Now, this must be the finale," but it's not.

But then there's a long pause, everyone holds their breath, and suddenly it begins. There's more color and light and noise than you ever thought possible, and you're not even wondering if it's the finale because you're too caught up in the moment. That's kind of like an orgasm.

An orgasm is involuntary, like a reflex, which means you don't have control over it, and you won't have control over your body during an orgasm. Your body will tense up; you may moan or scream or squeal. It will be an important part of sex to be vulnerable enough to allow orgasm to happen, to allow the loss of control, and to trust your husband with seeing you like this. It will be delightful to him. It will increase your intimacy in marriage. Just let it all happen.

Also, because of a woman's anatomy, she may experience more than one orgasm. After a short period of relaxation following her first orgasm, if her husband resumes stimulation, she can come to orgasm again (often much more quickly and easily than before).

For some women, the first orgasm is always best. For others, multiple orgasms increase in intensity and pleasure. I highly recommend trying this out for yourself, to see if you enjoy multiple orgasms. However, your clitoris is incredibly sensitive during this time, so even the lightest pressure may be unbearable. You'll have to communicate well to your husband during this time, as what normally feels good to you may not be pleasurable anymore. Communicate and have a healthy curiosity to find what feels good enough to bring you to another orgasm.

A man will have only one orgasm. If you start to feel sorry for him here, remember that on the flip side, it's incredibly easy for him to orgasm, while it's harder for a woman. His body will tense up, he may moan or yell, and he will breathe heavily.

His orgasm is directly tied to the ejaculation of his sperm. The sperm will shoot out in pulses, about one to two seconds apart. These pulses are also related to his pleasure, so when it pulses, he feels pleasure. *didn't know that*

The orgasm phase can last anywhere from a couple of seconds to one minute.

The Resolution Phase

After an orgasm, there's an incredible release of tension and you feel more relaxed than you have ever felt before. You'll feel satisfied, content, happy, bonded to your husband, physically and emotionally at rest. The moments following an orgasm are an amazing part of sex.

This is a wonderful time to cuddle and rest with your spouse, not wanting anything. Perhaps talk about non-stressful or happy things. Do a recap of your lovemaking. Compliment each other. Affirm each other. Say, "I love you." Don't necessarily be in a hurry to get out of the moment. (If it's hard for you to stay put for too long without cleaning up, go to the bathroom and clean up, then come back to bed and enjoy the relaxed moment with your husband.)

The resolution phase solidifies the bonds that have been formed during sex. Cherish those special moments. Be careful and sensitive, encouraging and kind. You see a side of your husband here that no one else on earth will ever see. And he sees the same in you. Hold these moments with tender hands.

Four Surprising Things about Sex

I was prepared that sex wasn't going to be like it is in the movies. I knew it was going to be slightly awkward and things wouldn't go as smoothly as I had hoped. However, I think I may have been over prepared for it to be terrible. Instead of having any hope that it would be romantic and intimate, I was so focused on the negative that it took me a few weeks to start remembering that sex is a fun and enjoyable thing too.
—Rose

Having sex for the first time, or having sex with your husband for the first time, will be a completely new and fresh experience, loaded with excitement and adventure. You won't know what to expect, but in my interviews with women, there were four things that they found particularly surprising about sex:

Sex Is Fun

In our culture, sex is often portrayed as serious or even dangerous, but in real-life relationships, sex is often described as fun! It's a place to be silly and to laugh, to be playful and curious, lighthearted and joyful. Many, many women talk about how they love to laugh with their husbands during sex, making jokes and letting loose. "Sex is the most important form of adult play,"[24] and when you find yourself naked and vulnerable in front of another person, yet truly accepted and loved by that person, you suddenly have the buoyancy and joy of a child.

Sex Is Messy

Many people are surprised when they find out how messy sex can be. Your body will produce its own lubrication, natural oils, and liquid. You may use synthetic lubricant, which can be oily. When he orgasms, he will eject semen. All of this has to go somewhere, so if it's all in your vagina, it will come out. But even though you will be messy, you will not be dirty. Both a woman's and a man's bodily fluids are sterile and clean. In fact, they're so clean you could eat them and it wouldn't harm your body. Let yourself relax into the messiness, perhaps even seeing it as a playful element of sex.

Sex Is Hard Work

Grace says, "It took a lot of practice before we could both orgasm during sex. Sometimes it felt like work. And sometimes we would try so long and so hard to get me to orgasm, and if it didn't happen, I would feel so defeated. However, we kept at it, and when we started to figure things out and find more and more success, it felt like we had overcome the obstacle together, and we took a lot of pride in it." Many people assume that satisfying sex comes naturally, but it's actually a skill that you acquire through lots of hard work and practice. This is why many couples admit to experiencing better sex the longer they've been married! Keep on working at it, and don't give up! It will get better!

Sex Is Better for Your Husband When You Enjoy Yourself

Many women were surprised to find just how much their husbands cared about their wife's sexual pleasure. Nora said, "I learned that a lot of my husband's enjoyment during sex depends upon how much I enjoy it. The more he is able to please me, the more he is pleased!" These women found that the way to selflessly satisfy their husbands during sex was to be utterly satisfied themselves. Crazy, huh? Give yourself the freedom to explore the things that make you happy during sex, and then make sure to let your husband know how great he makes you feel.

Sexual Hygiene

We clean up immediately after. I've never been much of a
cuddler. It's like, way to go, high-five, good night!
—Iris

Proper hygiene is essential when having sex. Taking care of your body now has ramifications not only for your own well-being but also for that of your husband. As Paul says in Ephesians, "Husbands ought to love their wives as they love their own bodies. For a man who loves his wife actually shows love for himself. No one hates his own body but feeds and cares for it, just as Christ cares for the church" (Eph. 5:28–29 NLT). So a wife not only cares for her own body, but also for her husband's, as a way to mimic the service of Christ for his church.

Both a wife and her husband should wash and dry their genitals on a regular basis. As discussed in Part One, you don't need anything other than water to do this properly. Drinking lots of water and quickly changing out of wet or sweaty clothes will also help prevent infection.

After sex, you and your husband should urinate, flushing out your systems. Then wash your genitals, taking great care to clean all of your exterior genitalia. (A woman need not clean her vagina, as it is self-cleaning.) Finally, dry off completely—bacteria thrives in a warm, moist environment.

Do not have sex if either of you have an infection of any kind, but especially a urinary tract infection or a yeast infection. Also, don't engage in any kind of sexual intercourse if either of you has any cuts or sores on your genitalia.

As Dr. Fogarty says, "Your body is a temple, and it's made to glorify God. So you have to keep it clean, and you have to cherish it."

8

Understanding Sexual Arousal

I think the best advice I was given was from my husband. He told me to do whatever I needed, or move however I wanted, to make it feel good for myself, because anything I did felt good to him. It gave me the freedom to explore new ways that made it good for me, knowing that he was having a good time and enjoying it just as much.

—Bethany

God will hold us accountable for every permitted pleasure that we forfeit.

—The Talmud

Sexual arousal is both instinctive and mysterious. It's something you can't help feeling, yet struggle to describe. And sometimes it's elusive, harder to grasp than a cloud. In this chapter, we'll examine female arousal—the unique qualities of female sexuality, how to feel sexual pleasure, and what to do when you don't—as well as the basics of male arousal and how to give pleasure to your husband.

Female Arousal

*The strangest paradox in the realm of sexuality is the
widespread idea that a woman's orgasmic capability is less
than a man's, whereas in reality it may be even greater.*
—Tim and Beverly LaHaye

God has created in every woman the potential for a natural and flourishing orgasmic ability. Whatever you may have heard, whatever you may have read, a woman can experience satisfying and complete sexual encounters with her husband, especially if she is familiar with erogenous zones and clitoral orgasms.

Erogenous Zones

Erogenous zones are places on your body that, when touched, can create a sexual response. For example, if your husband were to come up behind you, slip his hand up your shirt, and cup your breast, there's a pretty good chance you would have a sexual feeling of some kind. You will most likely have a strong sexual response like this to any touching of your breasts and genitals (the same is true for men).

However, there are other erogenous zones. Think about when he lays his hand on the small of your back, whispers something in your ear, or strokes your cheek. Most likely you're thinking that these things would feel good, romantic, or exciting. That's because the small of your back, your earlobe, and your face are all erogenous zones; also, your scalp, your neck, your mouth, your armpits (and breasts), your stomach, inner thighs, and the top of your bottom.

All of these areas contain the potential for sexual response, and it can feel so good for a couple to spend time caressing, touching, or massaging these areas, whether it's in public (a gentle hand on the neck) or in private (making out).

Even further, there is a sense in which all of your skin is an erogenous zone. I'm sure this isn't a surprise, though. I can remember when I was single that if I liked someone, all he would have to do was brush against my arm as we walked and I would get tingles up my spine!

If you pay attention to your erogenous zones, spend time touching his and have him touch yours, and experiment to find the places that you love the best, your sexuality will blossom!

Clitoral Orgasms

Probably the greatest sexual misconception is that the vagina is the seat of sexual feeling for a woman. If a man enters her vagina with his penis, she is expected to orgasm easily, quickly, and explosively or she is considered to have difficulty orgasming. But truly, that would be a physical impossibility for one simple reason—the vaginal wall contains very few nerve endings!

All women should shout a prayer of thanks to God for this fact; otherwise, we would die of pain if or when we delivered a child. Can you imagine how tortuous birthing a baby would be if we had sensitive nerve endings all over our vagina? Instead, God gave us a clitoris, an organ at the opening of our vagina to give us pleasure, which is stimulated during sex but not during birth. Hallelujah!

Clitoral orgasms are extremely accessible to every woman. Either your husband's hand or your own can touch, caress, and stroke your clitoris to create some unbelievable sensations. Or your husband can use his mouth to kiss, lick, and tickle your clitoris. I'm sure you're beginning to suspect how amazing this would feel. And if you are having intercourse, make sure that whatever position you're in, you're getting some good contact on your clitoris, whether it's against your husband's body or with the use of a hand.

Couples run into problems when they assume that the best way to have sex is when a woman orgasms during vaginal intercourse. And while intercourse can be incredibly satisfying—both you and your husband getting pleasure out of a simultaneous act, coming together to form one body–this idea can get a lot of people in trouble. Dr. Alex Comfort makes the point, "Saying that a woman 'should' climax with penetration is equivalent to saying that a man 'should' climax through having his testicles pulled. Some do, some don't, and in any case each to their own."[25]

If you and your husband concentrate attention on your clitoris, you will soon experience easy, quick, and explosive orgasms.

How to Get Turned On

Even though God created your body to be able to have an orgasm, this doesn't mean that it will come easily. An orgasm can be a tricky little thing for a woman. But God doesn't create anything poorly, and while a woman's orgasms can be elusive, he also created them to be magnificent, varied, and numerous.

If you're struggling to have an orgasm, have patience with yourself. You may feel pressure to perform for your husband or be impatient to experience sexual release. But don't worry, you'll figure it out eventually! Think of learning to orgasm as a journey. I imagine a woman with a determined expression on her face, wearing a flannel shirt and a backpack laden with gear, setting off on a trail leading over a mountain. It will take time, she may become tired or discouraged, but if she never gives up and keeps going in the right direction, eventually she'll reach that mountain peak.

Here are some tips for the journey of becoming more orgasmic:

1. Think about Sex
It takes time for a woman to become aroused, and some women will spend the whole day thinking about making love to their husbands that night. One woman even writes "T.S." in random places around her house to remind herself to "think sex."

Think about the way sex feels—warm, tingly, comforting, and exciting. Think about your love for your husband—the way he looks, his unique personality, and special memories from your past. Think about your husband's love for you—what he does to express his love for you, how he chose you out of all the women on earth, and how he wants to be with you. These thoughts will create a building sexual tension that will make you yearn for your husband.

2. Tackle Your Obstacles
If you're having trouble getting turned on, consider what may be getting in the way. Is there a lack of privacy that's distracting you? Do you feel too tired to have sex? Are you on a medication that's affecting your sex drive? Anti-depressants

Once you can pinpoint the obstacle, talk to your husband about it, and brainstorm ways to overcome it. Get a lock for your door. Have sex in the morning. Talk to your doctor about finding another prescription. You have a lot to gain from tackling these obstacles—you will enjoy sex more fully and your husband will appreciate the effort you put into your sex life.

3. Introduce Helpful Tools
There are some very helpful tools for achieving orgasm. Many women talk about the importance of relaxing when it comes to sexual arousal. Sip on a glass of wine or a mug of hot tea, light some candles, or take a bath. Even during the act of sex itself, remind yourself to relax into the moment, allowing yourself to feel the sensations in your body and letting your mind release into the love of your husband.

Other women need stimulation when it comes to sexual arousal. Make a playlist of romantic songs and listen to it throughout the day. Buy a vibrator or a vibrating ring to help stimulate sexual feeling on your clitoris during sex. Soaking in a warm bath and running water over your clitoris before sex can also produce a surge of sexual feeling.

It must be noted that these tools should never be used as a form of self-gratification. Remember that the goal is not to feel good, but rather to become more intimate with your husband.

4. Process Difficult Emotions

Negative emotions can deeply impact your sex drive. Anything from past sexual abuse to a current frustrating conflict can put a damper on your sex drive, or even completely extinguish it! Don't underestimate the power of emotions to affect the physical body, and be willing to commit to your own emotional health.

Find ways to process difficult emotions by journaling, praying, talking with a trusted friend, or going to therapy. It will take time and might even be painful to deal with these feelings, but only by getting honest with ourselves about the brokenness in our lives can we open ourselves up to the healing that God can provide.

5. Make yourself pretty

Taking some time to make yourself look or—more importantly—feel pretty can do wonders to turn you on. Give yourself thirty minutes in the bathroom. Soak in the tub. Shave. Put on lotion and perfume and creatively plan what you're going to wear. Let this be a relaxing experience, not motivated by some kind of burden to look a certain way for your husband, but rather as an opportunity to feel your best. God made a woman's form so beautiful and pleasing that it can even be pleasant to look at yourself!

The main point with all of these tips is to pay attention to your body and your mind. What would feel good? What is causing pain? What do you need to feel more sexually aroused? No one can answer these questions except for you! This is definitely a challenge, but think of achieving orgasm as an adventure. You're going to make a discovery about yourself, but you will have to be brave, strong, and persevering enough to make the journey.

To Orgasm or Not to Orgasm

The question of whether or not to orgasm during sex is very personal, and people have strong opinions either way. Sometimes, you simply can't orgasm. There are a number of reasons why this may occur.

At the beginning of marriage, it may be difficult to achieve orgasm, even if both you and your husband are working hard for you to reach climax. It may be impossible to orgasm if you are experiencing pain during sex. You may not be able to reach orgasm because you're on a certain medication that makes it difficult. You may have trouble having an orgasm if you're pregnant.

There will be other times when you choose not to orgasm because you don't want to. Orgasms can take a lot of effort on the part of a woman, and there are times when it doesn't seem worth it. If your husband has a much higher sex drive than you, it can be helpful to have a "quickie," where you help him to reach orgasm but you don't feel the need to orgasm yourself. Perhaps you enjoy meeting his needs in this way.

Because intimacy, not orgasm, is the goal of sex, there will definitely be moments when orgasm does not occur, and this is completely and totally okay.

As explained in *A Celebration of Sex: A Guide to Enjoying God's Gift of Sexual Intimacy* by Dr. Douglas Rosenau, Christian sex therapist Christopher McCluskey has created a more relational view of sex that emphasizes something called apex instead of the Orgasm Phase. Dr. Rosenau says, "It takes a mature person to understand that the emotional center of the apex is not orgasm, but a surrender to feelings and to each other. The term apex is purposefully used to de-emphasize chasing orgasms and to emphasize the deeper idea of abandonment and achieving a deeper oneness. Most often there will be that exciting climax, but there will be some times when an orgasm will not occur and yet an apex is achieved. Mature, older couples have often grown into this level of apex and enjoy its beauty. Souls have surrendered and joyful sexual-peak experiences are achieved, though no orgasm has occurred."[26]

However, a word of warning: when God created sex, he created a natural sexual progression that ends in orgasm. He gave both men and women this ability, and we should act accordingly. Sex is a mutual activity to be done between two people, and it's best when both men and women are participating fully. So, if you can't orgasm, continue practicing at sex until you and your husband are able to orgasm during a sexual encounter. This is something that God wants for you!

Additionally, make sure that when or if you choose not to orgasm, it's not because you're checking out of sex. Sometimes women can say things like, "I'm fine!" or "Don't worry about me," and while we are very good at serving our husbands selflessly, this can become a way for us to keep up our defenses, to not have to ask for help, to not let go of control, and to not put ourselves in a position where we need to ask our husbands for patience, service, and total acceptance.

Dr. Rosenau goes on to state, "Apexes cannot be reached without letting go, which is built on a series of individual choices. I will choose to trust; I will choose to feel; I will choose to give up control in front of and to my mate. It is interesting that many couples can create orgasms but not an apex because there are too many fears and walls to deep intimacy and trust. Let God help you surrender to Him and to each other on important nonsexual levels. This can create the foundation for sexual surrender."[27]

So even if you choose not to orgasm, perhaps adopt this concept of apex, so that you always allow sex to bring you closer to your husband. Never let the decision of whether or not to orgasm keep you from letting go of your own control, pride, or insecurity in exchange for a chance to grow closer to your husband.

Male Arousal

It can be fun that your husband is an easy read . . . You have a
lot of power in a fun, sexual way because he responds so
predictably.
                                              —Dr. Douglas Rosenau

Every man is different, and it will be an important, bonding, and no
doubt surprising journey to discover what pleases your husband.
However, here are a few points about male arousal that are true for
most men:

Men Are Visual

This well-known fact often leads women on a quest to find the perfect
lingerie or lipstick, but actually it just means that your husband wants
to see you naked; no matter what your body type, scars, curves, or
lumps, he will enjoy seeing and touching your naked body. Trust him
when he says he loves your body. Allow him to bask in the beauty of the
body God gave you.

This might also mean that he will favor positions in which he can
see you while making love to you. While a woman often closes her eyes
during sex, a man will like to soak in the beauty of his wife.

Men Appreciate Firm, Fast Movement

When it comes to movement, men usually appreciate a firmer, faster
thrust than we do. So whether you're performing oral sex, giving him a
hand job, or taking the lead in thrusting, he'll most likely want a pretty
rapid crescendo to a strong, hard thrust. Also, while women often like
variety and a change of pace, this can be disconcerting or frustrating to
a man. It will probably feel better for him if your pace remains steady.

At the same time, be gentle. A man's penis and testicles are incredibly sensitive. Be careful when holding and touching them. Be gentle, but firm.

Men Orgasm Quickly

On average, men orgasm with two minutes of consistent stimulation, whereas women take much longer.[28] This doesn't mean that men are too eager any more than it means that women aren't good at sex. It's simply a reflection of the differences that God designed in men and women. It's also an opportunity to overcome differences in order to come together in service and unity.

Give him grace if he orgasms quickly, but work with him to help him last. A firm, fast thrust will quickly bring him to climax, so change the speed of your thrusting to slow down his arousal. Change positions if he nears orgasm or let him bring you to orgasm before he becomes too deeply aroused. Practice together until he can last long enough for you to orgasm so that you can both have a complete sexual experience every time you come together.

Men Need Your Help

Like many newlyweds, Megan soon realized the importance of communication. She confessed, "Being really open and transparent at the beginning was tricky. We went into it really informed. We both had fairly realistic expectations, but I was expecting that everything between us was going to be completely understood. Instead, I needed to figure out what I wanted and to be able to communicate that to him and not just expect him to sweep me off my feet." I urge you to take Megan's words to heart and commit to communicating to your husband.

Make sure he's aware that a woman's sexual arousal takes ten times longer than a man's. Introduce him to the basics of female anatomy, and tell him about the importance of the clitoris for female arousal. Moan, sigh, or use words during sex when something feels great, and redirect the situation if he does something you don't like. Don't assume he knows what to do, and don't assume he doesn't care about your own satisfaction. Felicity says, "Sex that pleases a woman pleases a man too. I wanted to better understand my body and how to heighten my response to my husband, so I researched it. Next, I told my husband exactly what I had learned, and we figured it out from there."

Help him out by clearly communicating your perspective of your love life!

9

The Four Kinds of Sex

*I was absolutely clueless as to how to please my husband. I had
no idea how to give a hand job or a blow job, or what
movements felt good for him during sex. Thankfully, this just
meant more practice, which made him happy. Also, it's not like
the alternative would've been good for either of us. I'm glad I
was inexperienced in this arena. I just thought maybe I
would've had better instincts!*
                                    —Elizabeth

*Some men know that a light touch of the tongue, running from
a woman's toes to her ears, lingering in the softest way possible
in various places in between, given often enough and sincerely
enough, would add immeasurably to world peace.*
                                    —Marianne Williamson

I used to teach sex education to middle schoolers in the public school
system. As part of our curriculum, we taught each student that there
are four kinds of sex:

- *Vaginal Sex* (sex, intercourse)—when his penis is inserted into
your vagina

- *Manual Sex* (hand job, fingering)—when either of you uses your hand to stimulate the other's genitals
- *Oral Sex* (blow job, fellatio, cunnilingus)—when either of you use your mouth to stimulate the other's genitals
- *Anal Sex*—when either of you stimulates or penetrates each other's anus with your fingers or genitals.

Honestly, a big part of why we taught about these four different types of sex to students is because when they are told not to have sex, they sometimes think that oral sex, mutual masturbation and anal sex are not included. Our goal was to keep them from participating in these activities.

However, there's a strange irony. It's as though we tell kids, "There is more than one form of sex," but then when we get married, we forget that there is more than one form of sex! These are legitimate, natural forms of sex that can be very enjoyable to a married couple.

Not only that, but some of these other forms of sex will become absolutely essential to have in your repertoire. Remember that only one third of women can orgasm during vaginal sex, which means everyone else is using oral sex or mutual masturbation to get to the orgasm phase.

As a side note, because of your past or the way these other forms of sex have been talked about by Christians, their very nature may seem sinful or dirty. Please consider the fact that God does not condemn any of them. Think about the Song of Songs, a beautiful and erotic poem contained in the Bible! The sex life depicted in the poem is passionate, creative, and shockingly free from shame. In poetic language, the two lovers speak openly of their attraction, of their arousal, of their sensual touch of each other's bodies, and of the very act of sex.

He
How beautiful you are, my darling!
Oh, how beautiful!

Your eyes behind your veil are doves

. . . .

Your breasts are like two fawns,
like twin fawns of a gazelle
that browse among the lilies.
Until the day breaks
and the shadows flee,
I will go to the mountain of myrrh
and to the hill of incense.
You are altogether beautiful, my darling;
there is no flaw in you.

. . . .

She
Awake, north wind,
and come, south wind!
Blow on my garden,
that its fragrance may spread everywhere.
Let my beloved come into his garden
and taste its choice fruits.

. . . .

My beloved is radiant and ruddy,
outstanding among ten thousand.

. . . .

His lips are like lilies
dripping with myrrh.
His arms are rods of gold
set with topaz.
His body is like polished ivory
decorated with lapis lazuli.
—Song of Songs 4:1–5:14 NIV

If you study carefully, these verses are talking about mutual masturbation, oral sex, and vaginal sex. These are pure, God-given ways to enjoy and to grow intimate with your spouse. "God's plan is for us to pursue and know him in and through the sexual intimacy we have with our spouses. . . God is a God of passion. He adores joy, and he delights in our delight in glory. . . Eroticism is God's playful creation, his delight in delighting the erogenous heart of his creatures."29

When it comes to pure, godly sex, anything is allowed, as long as it's not extramarital (adultery, threesomes, porn, etc.). Seriously, anything is allowed! Let the Lord retrain your brain so that you think of sex not as dirty but as delightful. Oral sex? Awesome. Sensual massage? Great! Taking naked pictures of each other? Do it! When you're in a private place with your husband, let yourself be curious and free. Let the bonds of guilt and the lies of Satan fall off your heart, and learn what it means to participate in this amazing gift of God.

Vaginal Sex

For the first several months of marriage I don't think we did anything but missionary style. And I didn't even know women did anything but lie there during sex. Isn't that awful!? I would have never had my first orgasm if it weren't for reading about different positions and ways that you can be stimulated.

—Molly

Vaginal sex is when your husband's erect penis is inserted into your vagina. It's the essence of sexuality, the coming together of two genders in love, serving each other on an emotional, spiritual, and physical plane, with the ultimate outcome being a sensation of total pleasure, contentment, and oneness and the possibility of the creation of a child.

Physically, vaginal sex feels good because of friction. In other words, if he puts his penis inside you and then both of you just lie there, it's not going to do anything for you. So you create friction by thrusting the penis back and forth within your vagina. While the friction does produce sexual pleasure, you'll want to use plenty of lubricant to soften the skin and prevent chafing. *never needed any*

Women have the best experience during vaginal intercourse when they employ lots of foreplay and know two key sex positions.

Foreplay

When a woman becomes aroused, her clitoris expands, much like a man's penis. This means the head gets bigger, more sensitive as well as more visible from the outside. Also, her vaginal opening expands. That tiny little tube that she may struggle to get a tampon into will open wider and wider until it's several times its original size. Also, her body secretes fluid during arousal—in much the same way that a man ejaculates semen—both before and during orgasm.

[handwritten margin note: news to me]

When I started having sex, I had no idea that a woman's sexual response was so similar to a man's. I guess you don't think about it since a woman's arousal is mostly internal. But I have this little theory. No couple would dream of beginning intercourse before his penis was enlarged and hard enough to get into her. However, I think that lots of couples start intercourse before a woman's vaginal opening is fully enlarged or her clitoris is properly swelled. It's hard to blame them, since her genitals aren't visible. What ends up happening is that because the opening is too small and she hasn't secreted enough fluid to lubricate her vagina, besides the pain of the chafing, there's no way she can feel pleasure because her clitoris isn't even big enough to be touched by the penis!

All sex therapists and premarital counselors worth their salt will mention this to some degree. They'll say, "Use foreplay," "Make out," "Use his hand to help you reach climax," but they often don't tell you why. It's not that a woman likes kisses more than she likes sex. The real point is that she can't like sex before she has kisses.

And the truth is, it doesn't work the other way. I mean, he can come into you. But it will hurt and feel unnatural and you won't be able to engage, which isn't God's intention for you. God wants both of you to be mutually satisfied by each other, so don't skip your own sexual arousal!

Positions

Because you can't have an orgasm without stimulating your clitoris, and because your clitoris is outside your body (not in your vagina where the penis is during sex), sex positions become a big deal for a woman.

For example, the doggy position (when you are on hands and knees and he inserts his penis from behind you) makes it impossible to orgasm because nothing is rubbing on your clitoris. Thankfully, there are two great positions for having an orgasm during intercourse.

use your own hands

The first position is with you on top. This can be a good position because you're in control of the movements. You can wriggle and move and tilt and push until you find the right feeling. Also, your husband will love this position because he can see your beautiful body the whole time.

The second is with him on top and with your hips elevated. It doesn't work unless your legs are in the air or you put a pillow under your hips. Once my husband and I figured out this position, we called it the Magic Button. It just worked every time.

You'll still have to experiment and practice a lot in these two positions before figuring out how to orgasm. (Also, depending on your own anatomy, these positions may not work.) However, besides rare occurrences, these are the only two positions in which a woman can have an orgasm during intercourse without direct stimulation of the clitoris. *never orgasmed during sex*

Vaginal intercourse is the bread and butter of sex. Dr. Alex Comfort remarks that "the symbolism alone makes it central to the whole performance."[30] There's something about intertwining your bodies, coming together as one, and feeling every movement at the same time as you pleasure and serve each other. In fact, it's so pleasurable that even some women who don't orgasm during vaginal intercourse still consider it a favorite way to make love. *so close*

kinda scary cus you are on display, must be very confident

116

Manual Sex

*Our premarital counselor said that in the beginning, when
you're trying to figure things out, it can become all about the
dude. So we decided that we would start, then my husband
would touch me until I finished, then he would climax.*

—Eva

Manual sex is when you use your hand to stimulate your partner's genitals. This is an incredibly important element of sex. We've already talked about how "handy" it can be, when trying to orgasm, for your husband to use his hand to stimulate your clitoris, but it's also an enjoyable act for you to perform on your husband as well. Remember that this isn't about rules, but about enjoying each other's bodies and finding ways to lovingly serve each other by making each other feel amazing physically. hand job :)

yes!

Receiving Manual Sex

You will experience a pleasant sensation when he uses his hand or the tips of his fingers to gently massage your clitoris, vulva, or the inside of your vagina. He can stroke up and down, rub in a circular motion, "tickle," or whatever feels good. Use natural oils (coconut oil, olive oil, etc.) or artificial lubricants to soften the skin and smooth the massaging movements.

Communicate often and clearly. Whenever something feels good, say, "That feels good." Whenever something doesn't feel good, ask, "Can you try something else?" You can communicate in other ways besides talking too. Feel free to moan or sigh (or scream!) to communicate your pleasure.

It may feel good for him to insert one or two fingers into your vagina while stimulating your clitoris. Ask him to sort of "hook" his fingers up into your vagina, pressing on the "top" of your vaginal wall.

g-spot

As he explores this area, you may discover that it feels especially good. If not, let him know. At least you tried!

Try touching your husband while he is giving you a hand job. Caress his hair, rub his shoulders, or manually stimulate his penis. However, if it's too hard to concentrate, just lie there and enjoy it.

If he brings you through the orgasm phase with manual stimulation, let him know when you're orgasming (either with words or vocalization) and then let him know when you're through. If he continues to stimulate you, it will feel uncomfortable on your extra-sensitive clitoris.

Giving Manual Sex

Remember that men generally like firm, constant stimulation. Also, they tend to like fast movements. Listen to his feedback. If he's not communicating, ask him questions about what feels good. His penis and scrotum are incredibly sensitive, so remember to be gentle and try not to bend or hit his genitals accidentally when you're making fast thrusts.

Women are skilled at multitasking, so you might find your mind is a mile away while you give him a hand job. I encourage you to engage your mind in the action. Think about your husband and how he must be feeling. Let your eyes soak up his body and concentrate on what you love about him. Perhaps you can straddle his leg or do something that stimulates your clitoris so that you can stay aroused during the process. Or ask him to give you a hand job at the same time! (However, this can be difficult to pull off for both of you simultaneously.) Try to stay engaged. After all, this is sex, a time for intimacy and love, not crafting a grocery list in your head.

If you stimulate him through the orgasm phase, have a plan for when he ejaculates. Perhaps neither of you mind the mess, so let it happen. Or you may prefer to do it in the bathroom, in the shower, or over the sink. Or maybe you have a towel nearby and you lay it across his pelvis to catch what comes out. But you'll want to have a plan.

Manual sex is especially fun and helpful during the first few months of sex. It can be a relatively simple or easy way to come to the orgasm phase, and it's also an important way to learn about each other's bodies and to watch and observe what happens to each other throughout the different phases of sex.

Oral Sex

On our first night together, my husband's penis was the first one I had ever seen up close. It shocked me. I actually starting laughing because I was so embarrassed. When we had sex, I could never think about his penis because I thought it was ugly and really weird. And I thought my vagina was even weirder . . . But then one night my husband did oral sex. I was shocked that he wanted to touch me down there with his mouth. But seeing how much he loved me and loved my body, I started looking at his differently. I began to love it. Every curve, every muscle, and every bit of his penis. Now I love kissing it, and we do oral sex all the time. Now when I think about his penis, I get in the mood!

—Zoe

Oral sex is when you caress your partner's genitals with your mouth. It's sex, just as vaginal intercourse is sex, but there are so many things in our culture that have warped oral sex into an act that feels dirty, obscene, or oppressive. But we don't have to let our culture define sex. We can pray and ask God to retrain our hearts and minds to see all kinds of sex as good, godly, fun, freeing, and beautiful.

Instead of giving or receiving oral sex because you feel pressured or because you're afraid your husband will be disappointed in you if you don't, I suggest letting it happen more organically. During sex, touch his whole body. Let your hands roam free, doing whatever feels good to you. (Did you catch that? Touch him in ways that feel good to you.) Kiss him all over. Kiss his mouth, his eyes, the indenture right behind his ears. Kiss his broad chest and his fingers. Kiss his penis.

Let yourself explore and grow comfortable with his body. Find out how his body turns you on. What about him do you find erotic? Don't think of anything but your body, your husband's body, and what feels good to both him and you. Now can you see how oral sex could happen on its own?

Allow all of this action to take place vice versa. Let him touch and caress you. Let him explore your body, delighting in the way you look and feel. Let him watch your face as he does this. Release yourself into the joy of these moments.

There are no rules for oral sex. However you do it is perfect. Below are some tips that you may find helpful, but if something isn't helpful, tell yourself that it must've been a bad tip and forget about it.

Giving Oral Sex

Cleanliness is important, so ask him to take a shower or wash himself beforehand. You may like to rub honey or coconut oil on him beforehand. The coconut oil is a good lubricant, the honey is anti-bacterial, and they both taste and smell good. This is especially helpful if the smell or taste of his penis bothers you.

You can have oral sex in any position, but start with him lying on the bed. This seems to be extra comfortable. Don't think that you have to go from the Excitement Phase all the way to the Orgasm Phase doing oral sex. Do it as long as you want or can and then move on to other kinds of sex.

Cover the base of his penis with your hand, and put only the top third in your mouth. Suck on the end of his penis, perhaps closing your throat with your tongue to prevent a gag reflex. Suck over and over again, building pressure and friction. Or kiss and lick his penis all over.

He may like for you to gently but firmly cup his testicles with your hand while you give oral sex. Also, the vein that runs along the length of his penis on the bottom is very sensitive, as are the tip and the ridge where the head meets the shaft, so it can feel especially good for him if you work these areas.

Ask your husband to let you know before he orgasms so that you have time to pull away. If you are interested in letting him orgasm during oral sex, then go for it! It may feel good to him if you suck whenever you feel his penis spasm during climax, to make the sensation more intense. (Every man's semen tastes different. If you do get a taste of your husband's semen, try to figure out what it tastes like. Is it salty? Sweet? It may be fun to tell him what you're thinking.)

Receiving Oral Sex

What they eat

Many women encounter trouble receiving oral sex. Perhaps you think that your vagina is gross, or that it smells bad, or maybe you can't relax enough to find pleasure. If this is the case, pray about it. Tell God how you feel and ask him to help you think about sex the way he does (your body is wonderfully made, your vagina is clean, and sex in marriage is godly and good!). However, you never have to have sex in any way that makes you uncomfortable, and you shouldn't feel bad if oral sex isn't for you. *but you're missing out*

Spend some time beforehand to clean your vulva and to get yourself feeling your best. This is as much for your benefit as it is for your husband. Knowing that you are clean and presentable will help you to relax in the moment. You may wish to rub coconut oil or honey on your vulva and labia so that your skin is moist and relaxed, and so that you know you smell good.

Once your husband starts, be sure to communicate. He will appreciate the guidance. Even if you're not sure what you want, with practice and good communication, you'll both be able to figure out what feels good to you.

Remember to relax. This is probably the biggest barrier for women to receiving oral sex. Insecurity and anxiety will creep into your mind, but gently push them aside so that you can receive this love from your husband.

Charlotte tells this moving account of her first attempt at oral sex: "One of our most intimate moments was when we didn't have intercourse at all. I performed oral sex for the first time. Afterward, we were just lying there on the kitchen floor, and it was just a really cool moment because I knew that he felt accepted by me completely. And that's what the gospel is, I think: that you're totally accepted. It was really awesome because I felt so close to him. I would've never thought that this would be the best sex because I didn't personally experience anything that felt really good physically, but I just remember thinking that it was so awesome."

Anal Sex ouch!

While this is also a legitimate form of sex, you should exercise extreme caution when having anal sex for two reasons. One, there is a heightened risk of infection because of the presence of bacteria in the anus. Secondly, and most importantly, the anal lining is thinner than the vaginal lining and runs the risk of tearing. It is possible to inflict permanent damage to a woman's anus during anal sex. Because of the health risks, I advise researching anal sex if either of you are interested in trying it. Understand anatomy, proper hygienic practices associated with anal sex, and the emotional status of each partner before experimenting with anal sex.

Experimenting

Know that the bed isn't the only place and night isn't the only time.

—Mila

Even though this whole chapter can seem like a list of dos and don'ts, know that there isn't such a thing as a "right way" to have sex. God intended sex to be an arena of creativity, playfulness, and wonder, so let yourself "break the rules" in order to have fun with your husband. Try lots of different positions, not only the ones mentioned here. Spend an hour on foreplay, stretching the sexual tension to its breaking point, or have no foreplay at all, rushing a "quickie" in order to have a moment of intimacy before you leave for work.

Many women shared about the joy they have found in creative expressions of sexuality with their husbands. One couple shares their sexual fantasies with each other and then work together to make them happen. A group of girlfriends formed an email thread in which they shared "recipes" for a night of great sex. Another couple was driving past a hotel in their suburban town and stopped on a whim, enjoying an hour of great sex on crisp white sheets. Another woman says that she and her husband designate one night a week as "Experiment Night," when they each suggest something new.

For some of us, "breaking the rules," experimenting, and creativity can seem nearly impossible in a place of such deep vulnerability. It's scary to open yourself up to your secret thoughts in full view of your partner, and it can be equally disconcerting to witness your husband's innermost desires when you're the only one who can fulfill them. But this is precisely the purpose of romantic love.

In her provocative book on married sexuality, Esther Perel writes, "Erotic intimacy is the revelation of our memories, wishes, fears, expectations, and struggles within a sexual relationship. When our innermost desires are revealed, and are met by our loved one with acceptance and validation, the shame dissolves. It is an experience of profound empowerment and self-affirmation for the heart, body, and soul." [31]

It's this dissolution of shame that is the pinnacle of sexual intimacy in marriage. It takes us back to the garden of Eden, the perfect expression of sex and marriage, when Adam and Eve lived together and "felt no shame" (Gen. 2:25 NLT). It's a trademark of godly sex, and we find it when we are both completely vulnerable and completely accepting of one another.

10

True Sex Appeal

There is no such thing as an ugly woman.
—Vincent Van Gogh

More important than your breast size, more important than your waist size, more important than the length of your legs is your attitude.
—Dr. Kevin Leman

confidence in the perfect original God made you

"How can I be good in bed?"

This is a question we all have, isn't it? I think in the end, that's the nagging question that often propels people to read magazines and books about sex and to watch sex scenes. How can I be good at sex? How can I give my husband pleasure? How can I make him feel awed by and satisfied in our love life?

Because of the uniqueness of each marriage relationship, it would be naive of me to try to answer this question for everyone, but I would like to challenge a common assumption and offer a few suggestions.

First of all, I think there's a stereotype of a woman who is "good in bed." It's the image of a tall, sultry woman showing up at a man's apartment wearing a trench coat (and only a trench coat), pushing him down on his bed, and climbing on top of him with a very serious expression on her face. She's mysterious and dangerous, and her personality doesn't exist outside of her sexuality. This works well for sexual relationships that aren't committed, where people don't know or understand each other's personalities, when the ultimate goal in sex is passion or thrill.

But God created sex to be so much more than that. He wanted two people to commit themselves to each other in lifelong love and service in order to grow to know each other—to truly know and be known. Intimacy is the goal, to be achieved through pleasure, community, covenant, and bonding. Because this is the case, there's a whole new way to be "good in bed." Instead, true sex appeal consists of warmth, humor, availability, initiative, communication, and vulnerability.

Warmth

Couples often look at me with surprise in the counseling office when I give them this homework: "I want you to go home and for the next two weeks, I want you to be nice to each other." I think this advice startles and resonates with them because it's a simple concept; but they know they have been neglecting this important skill of every great marriage.
—Dr. Douglas Rosenau

Honestly, I struggled to think of a word to describe this first attribute. I thought of words like kind, pleasant, easy to talk to, approachable, amiable, friendly, considerate, and affectionate. But my favorite word comes from a scene in The Office in which Michael asks Jim why he likes Pam. Jim says, "She's warm."[32]

A man isn't some weird, sex-crazed being who doesn't care who you are on the inside as long as you are supermodel-hot and have a vagina. Sex is emotional and personal for a man, and your response to him before, during, and after sex can have a profound effect upon him.

make or break him

If you're responsive, content, and warmhearted, he will drink you up like a tall glass of cold water. If you're sullen, resigned, unhappy, or discontent, no amount of lingerie can satisfy him.

Consider this heartfelt explanation from one husband: "A man really does feel isolated, even with his wife. But in making love, there is one other person in this world that you can be completely vulnerable with and be totally accepted and not judged. It is a solace that goes very deep into the heart of a man."[33]

Sex is emotionally powerful in the heart of a man, and your warmhearted attitude toward your husband makes him feel loved.

Humor

We've learned to laugh a lot when we have sex. That really
helps me, because I struggle with wanting to perform well for
him and to be sexy. The best sex we have is when we are both
laughing and feel intimately safe with each other.
—Penelope

A lot of the time, it will feel like sex is counterintuitive, like you just can't figure out the best way to do it without some outside advice. However, there's one instinct you have that will serve you well–the instinct to laugh. My friend Savannah says, "We learned early on that if something awkward or embarrassing happens, just laugh. Things like that are going to happen and you can't avoid it. You may as well enjoy those things instead of fear them."

As a newlywed, you may assume that laughter isn't sexy, that it ruins the moment. Nothing could be further from the truth! Take a moment to think about when your husband makes you laugh. Suddenly you feel happy inside, open toward him. It makes you like him more and endears you to him. Or consider when he laughs at your joke. It feels amazing, doesn't it? It's a kind of compliment, really. Laughter will bond you two together so quickly.

Laughter shoots endorphins through your body, causing feelings of happiness, contentment, and bonding. (Those are the same endorphins you get during an orgasm.)

Laughter can help to rid your sex life of feelings of guilt or dirtiness. People don't laugh with each other during a one-night stand. People don't laugh with each other during affairs. People laugh with each during holy, monogamous sex. It will clear the air, endear you to each other, and permeate the air with a feeling of purity and lightness.

Also, choosing to laugh instead of feeling offended or resentful is a beautiful way to be like Jesus. It's a way to smooth things over quickly and selflessly if one of you makes a mistake during sex.

Laughter is truly one of the best ingredients for amazing sex.

Availability

I am my lover's, and my lover is mine.
—Song of Songs 6:3 NLT

This poetic verse is a beautiful depiction of love. It conveys feelings both of ownership and sacrifice, and of receiving and giving. It's sort of intoxicating in its sensuality, don't you think? Oh, to feel so deeply about someone that you've given your body to him . . . and then to be loved so deeply in return that he gives his body to you!

There are several places in Scripture that teach this precept of marriage, but never is it so emotionally charged. Also, nowhere else is it so evident that this is a picture of Jesus and his church. Think about the extent to which Jesus has given himself to you. And then think about how, in your grateful love, you want to give yourself to Jesus.

The Lord is asking us to show the world a tangible picture of this: Jesus and his bride with skin on (see Eph. 5:22–33). There are many ways we give ourselves to our spouses, but in sex it's even more tangible, more literal than anywhere else. You literally give your body to your spouse and him to you, to do with what you will. It's a lovely depiction of trust, of humility, of service.

However, this doesn't work if you're faking it. "God loves a cheerful giver" (2 Cor. 9:7 ESV). It's the golden rule of giving. Sacrifice only means something if it's cheerful and authentic. Suppressed resentment and bitterness completely negate any "giving" that might have occurred and will poison your relationship with your husband. It's probably better to say no than to say yes and feel burdened or resentful.

Also, you don't have to say yes all the time. Be real with your husband and tell him if you're feeling tired or not in the mood. (Or ask him to "butter you up.") Marriage is about intimacy, and sometimes the most intimate thing you can do is transparently show him your selfishness or weakness. You won't be perfectly Christlike all the time. Again, don't fake it—that's hypocrisy.

And remember, you can expect your husband to be available to you too. Marriage and sex are a two-way street. While demanding sex is never acceptable, know that you *can* go to him with your burdens, with your worries and cares. Go to him when you need affection and affirmation. Go to him when you want sex. He's your husband, and God has put him in your life to protect and care for you. Whether that's through conversation, companionship, or sex, he is yours, just as you are his.

Initiative

*Don't always wait for your husband to initiate sex. Sometimes
you should be the one to reach over and pull him in for a long
kiss goodnight. And when you do, be ready to get it on!*
—Phoebe

Once, when Logan and I were dating, he came to me with a complaint.
"Whenever we hold hands," he said, "you don't hold my hand. You just
let your hand hang limp in mine. Don't you like holding hands?"

I was surprised by this. I loved walking everywhere hand in hand
and was completely unaware that I wasn't holding his hand. What I
realized was that I loved the feeling of being held so much, that I wasn't
even reciprocating the gesture. I was so completely satisfied with the
arrangement that I wasn't thinking about what it must feel like to him.

If you're a woman whose husband does most of the sexual
instigating in your relationship, this is something to keep in mind. It can
be so easy to take their initiative for granted, and even though we're
enjoying it, we may forget to give any verbal, physical, or relational cues
that we love it.

Like my hand-holding mistake, it's an easy fix. Instead, respond to
your husband's advances with verbal or physical signs of appreciation.
Or find a time to initiate sex yourself. This can be an opportunity for
you to dream a little and plan sex "your way." It will both delight and
enlighten your husband to witness your own sexual expression.

Vulnerability

*Vulnerability is not winning or losing; it's having the courage
to show up and be seen when we have no control over the
outcome.*
                                                    —Dr. Brené Brown

Women are often extremely intuitive when it comes to intimacy, and I think this will be a great area for you to tap into, feeling your way through sex with your husband, on a constant search for intimacy. However, vulnerability is one aspect of intimacy that can be very difficult for women.

Vulnerability is all about taking initiative, making the first move, showing weakness, and taking emotional risks. Dr. Brené Brown speaks of this kind of wholehearted love that says "I love you" first. It's a love that acts with no guarantees. It shows a willingness to invest in a relationship that may or may not work out.[34] Scary, right?

On days when this level of vulnerability and self-sacrifice seems impossible, remember the gospel. Remember that Jesus loved you and gave himself for you (see Gal. 2:20). Before there was any guarantee of your love for him, while you were still in the thick of sin, Jesus endured torment and death in order to bring you into oneness with himself. "The gospel can fill our hearts with God's love so that you can handle it when your spouse fails to love you as he or she should. That frees us to see our spouse's sins and flaws to the bottom—and speak of them—and yet still love and accept our spouse fully. And when, by the power of the gospel, our spouse experiences that same kind of truthful yet committed love, it enables our spouses to show us that same kind of transforming love when the time comes for it."[35]

Sex is all about letting go. In fact, you can't even have an orgasm without "letting go." It's about putting yourself in the weakest, most vulnerable position in front of someone else. It's about entrusting your body, emotions, and spirit to another person: to a man. You've done it in the act of covenantal vows, and now in sex you're doing it in a very physical, tangible way. You're letting him see your stretch marks, letting him touch the funny mole on your back, letting him hear you make noises you've never heard yourself make. You're asking him to do things for you that you can't do for yourself.

But herein lies the beauty of Christian marriage: he's making himself vulnerable to you too. That tough, strong man will also stand before you, naked, and ask you to love him just as he is. And like you, he does this even with the possibility of rejection. But when you're both being vulnerable with each other, when you both present yourselves to each other just as you are, then you have the freedom to fall into each other's arms. It's like a big, glorious, mutual trust fall. You catch each other and exult in the security of someone else who has seen you in your nakedness, heard your cry for intimacy, and answered "Yes!" Someone who wants you—all of you—for all eternity.

Personal Style

Before our honeymoon, I had read that it can be really sexy during a date to lift your foot between his legs and caress him under the table. But when I did this, my new husband was so uncomfortable. I've discovered since then that he's a private, modest person and likes sex best when we have utter privacy.
—Erin

In this chapter, I argue that "sexiness" is more than what Victoria's Secret would have you believe. I believe that things like warmth, humor, and availability can go a lot further when trying to set the mood and get it on with your spouse. However, appearances really do matter, and it would be a shame if we all decided to stop making ourselves look attractive (whatever that might be). Everyone has a personal style, and it's important to both know your own and that of your husband.

For example, maybe your husband doesn't care much for lacy garters and a room full of candles, but he loses his mind when you step out of the bedroom in a tight gray T-shirt. Or perhaps he appreciates your whispered sweet-nothings but gets frustrated when you make jokes during sex.

And don't forget yourself. Sometimes I wonder if lingerie isn't more important for women than it is for men; putting on a gorgeous dress made of lace and silk can be just the thing for getting in the mood! And maybe you don't care if your husband goes to the gym every day, as long as he's clean and smells good when he slips into bed with you at night.

In fact, it's kind of fun to find the quirky and personal things that your spouse finds sexual. Logan knows that I like his broad shoulders. I heard one woman go on and on about about how much she loved her husband's very hairy chest. A man I know asked his wife to never wear brown. All of these things have very little real value when it comes to finding your spouse attractive, but like sprinkles on a cake, they can add a fun element once you have the foundation in place.

With all that said, I would like to make one very important observation. My brother-in-law often tells his wife, "You're my type. And if you ever change, then so will my type." This is such a healthy way to understand attraction and harness your own sexuality for good. He's saying that he doesn't think of any woman besides his wife as being "his type." And he's also telling his wife that he will always foster attraction for her, even if her body or hair or personality changes.

So know your personal style, find out what's attractive to your husband, but always submit that to the good of your marriage.

11

How to Be a Darling When You're Married

Sex is complex. There's no getting around that. If it were simple and easy, it wouldn't be so good.
—Lexi

I had this idea that once we started having sex, every glance, every sight of each other naked, every cuddle or embrace would be sexy, would give me tingles or warm fuzzies or something. But that wasn't true. The endorphins wear off. I think that's kind of why God gave us sex. To give us something we get addicted to that forces us to partake in intimacy. Even when there aren't warm fuzzies, you can experience glorious intimacy with your partner, no matter how hard the day, how brutal the fight, how mundane the existence.
—Heidi

Chastity within marriage is just as important as when you're single or engaged. As you seek to paint an accurate picture of Christ and his church, married sexuality will involve two basic parts:

- *Covenant Faithfulness.* Chastity, now that you're married, involves being sexually and emotionally faithful to your husband. This can mean anything from not sleeping with another man to refraining from comparing your husband to another man or woman. Covenant faithfulness is about choosing to love your husband faithfully the way Christ has loved us.

- *Enjoying Sexual Intimacy.* Another way to be chaste is to fully partake in the gift of sex. You and your husband should have sex regularly, selflessly, and joyfully. Sex is uniquely given to marriage —God didn't intend it to happen in any other kind of relationship —so embrace the gift of sex and use it to build intimacy with your spouse and to glorify God.

In this chapter, we'll look at some obstacles to covenant faithfulness and enjoying sexual intimacy, as well as ways to overcome them.

Negative Emotions

Sexual satisfaction has less to do with the act, more to do with your heart.

—Summer

Emotions are a delightful aspect of each created person. Throughout the Bible, we find that God himself feels emotion, often deeply and passionately! It is good to feel joy, love, and surprise, and even difficult emotions like sadness, fear, and anger have an important part to play in our lives.

But many women feel completely helpless when it comes to understanding their emotions. They speak of emotions as a biological force that takes over and leaves them breathless and horrified, left to pick up the pieces of their outbursts. Here we'll look at three negative emotions that undermine the covenant faithfulness we wish to exemplify in our marriages.

Guilt

Many women spend years believing that sex is dirty or wrong, and they struggle with feelings of guilt once they enter into a sexual relationship in marriage. Although these feelings are common, they're based on lies. Sex with your husband is not bad, but something wonderful created by God and given to you. Let the distorted image of sex get out of your head, and "be transformed by the renewal of your mind" (Rom. 12:2 ESV).

Broken Expectations

Every woman brings expectations into a marriage, including expectations about what sex will or should be like. Many times, these expectations will be broken or unmet, and often it feels like your heart is breaking at the same time. I remember being shocked when, on our honeymoon night, my husband didn't want to cuddle while we slept. I didn't even realize I had the expectation of constant nightly snuggle time until it didn't happen. I was so disappointed that I cried myself to sleep.

The feelings were so intense because somewhere in my brain I had associated cuddling at night with an affectionate marriage and a healthy sex life. So even though we had those things, I didn't believe it since we weren't cuddling.

The only way to deal with expectations about sex is to gently let them go. Show grace to yourself and your husband as you each discover these expectations and learn to accept the reality of the situation.

Comparison

"Comparison is the thief of joy."[36] Nothing will steal joy and pleasure from your marriage more quickly than comparing yourself or your husband to someone else. You will be tempted to compare your sex life to a friend's marriage, to a movie you once saw, or to your own daydreams, but it will only lead to heartache. Remember that Jesus loves and accepts you as you are, and so you can extend that same unconditional love and grace to yourself and your husband.

What to Do about Your Negative Emotions

If you struggle with negative emotions, give yourself the time and space to work through what you're feeling.

1. Be Honest about Your Feelings

Journal or talk with a trusted friend about what it is you're actually thinking and feeling. Be honest, even if what you're thinking is embarrassing or wrong or scary.

2. Seek Out the Truth and Tweak Your Thinking

Again, with the help of journaling or a trusted friend, find out what's actually true. Have you formed any assumptions about the situation? Do you believe a lie? Are you remembering the event the way it truly happened? Once you've done this, tweak your thinking so that it fits with the truth.

3. Root Yourself in God's Love

When we are honest about our feelings and seeking the truth, it will produce "a fresh discovery of the mercy of God in the gospel. Not only does God not reject or punish us for being honest and transparent about our whole selves, but he actually accepts and loves us where we are."[37] Be a darling by never letting go of your identity as a woman deeply loved by God.

Remember, your emotions are not a bad thing, but something that God gave you. Rachel Jankovic writes about a powerful tool for understanding and controlling emotions:

We tell our girls that their feelings are like horses—beautiful, spirited horses. But they are the riders. We tell them that God gave them this horse when they were born, and they will ride it their whole life. . . . When our emotions act up, it is like the horse trying to jump the fence and run down into a yucky place full of spiders to get lost in the dark. A good rider knows what to do when the horse tries to bolt—you pull on the reins! Turn the horse's head! Get back on the path! . . . The goal is not to cripple the horse, but equip the rider. A well-controlled passionate personality is a powerful thing. That is what dangerous women are made of. But a passionate personality that is unbridled can cause a world of damage.[38]

Different Sex Drives

I hated myself that I had looked forward to something for so many years and then when it was "okay," I wanted nothing to do with it. I wanted to want sex, but it wasn't happening.
—Amelie

One of the most significant challenges that most couples face is the problem of differing sex drives. And to clarify, it's not always the man who wants the most sex. A friend of mine once remarked that it's about 50/25/25:

- For 50 percent of couples, the man has a higher sex drive.
- For 25 percent of couples, the woman has a higher sex drive.
- For 25 percent of couples, they each have a high sex drive.[39]

I find it fascinating how rare it is to find couples with a similar sex drive. But considering the differences in bodies as well as in past and present lifestyles, it makes sense. Sometimes I think that learning how to find true unity with someone different from you is the very point of sex! Here are some ways that other women have learned to find intimacy in the face of differing sex drives:

Find a Rhythm of Regular Sex

Even though you and your husband may have different ideas of how often you should be having sex, make sure you find a rhythm of regular sex. This could mean every day, once a week, or even less than that. But work toward regular sex. You may be tempted to compare your sex life to someone else's. If your husband wants to have sex every day and you hear about a couple who has sex once a week, don't make him feel guilty for his high sex drive. Learn to embrace your own rhythm and schedule.

Be Open to Change

You may go through seasons when everything turns upside down and suddenly you want sex and he doesn't (or vice versa). Grace shared that this was a very difficult experience in her marriage: "My husband had a big drop-off in his sex drive about four years into our marriage. It totally confused me and made me feel like I had done something wrong, then that something was wrong with me, then that something was wrong with him, and finally it just felt frustrating and upsetting." Things like stress, diet, sickness, and medications can all factor in to a change in libido, so know that it's completely natural for this to happen. It's a new season. Take a deep breath, communicate your needs to each other, and try to find a new rhythm.

Be Selfless

Sex is about him. (For him, sex is about you, but you can't worry about that.) Be like Jesus and give up your body for the sake of love and humility. Mia offers this encouragement, "You won't always be in the mood for it. Your partner may be in the mood, and sometimes the right thing to do is to be selfless. Turns out 90 percent of the time, you end up enjoying it, too!"

Here are some tips for when you're not in the mood for sex:

- Tell him that you're not in the mood and ask if you can postpone it until later (if so, make sure it's within twenty-four hours).
- Ask your husband to man the house while you go take a bath. As you soak and relax, ask God to give you desire for your husband.
- Spend a few minutes getting prettied up. Sometimes the act of cleaning up, and looking and smelling great, will turn you on.
- Just go for it (make sure to use lots of foreplay first so your body is ready) knowing that you'll end up enjoying the process.
- Communicate as much as possible about what you are feeling and ask him how he is feeling. If needed, seek counseling.

Some tips for when you want more sex than your husband:

- Start initiating sex. Don't wait for him to ask you.
- Be aware of your expectations and make appropriate changes to your thinking. Stop expecting your husband "to meet your sexual needs perfectly. Settle for improvement. The perfect sex life you have in your mind probably doesn't exist; it's far more helpful to work toward something that's better than to fight over an ideal two people will probably never achieve."[40]
- Comfort yourself with the truth that just because you have more libido than your husband, it doesn't mean you're not desirable to him.
- If you're dealing with feelings of suspicion or resentment toward your husband, pray about it and seek a godly mentor whom you can talk to.
- Communicate as much as possible about what you're feeling, and ask him how he is feeling. If needed, seek counseling.

When You Can't Have Sex

Don't stop making love; broaden your understanding of it.
− Dr. Douglas Rosenau

Even though enjoying regular sex is a way to be chaste in marriage, couples will encounter many instances when sex is difficult or impossible. You may have to go without sex during your period, when you or your husband travel for work, while visiting family and friends, or during times of sickness. When this happens, don't despair.

Remember That You Went without Sex for Many Years

You can go without sex for a couple days or weeks if you need to. The Lord will give you the self-control and strength you need. Pray and read his Word during this time to stay extra close to God.

Get Creative

In many cases, if you're creative and spontaneous, you can still have sex during these tricky times. For example, if you have visitors, be quiet and have cleanup handy so you don't have to make any naked runs to the bathroom. If you're sick or on your period, try something new that doesn't involve intercourse. Give each other massages, passionately make out, or have manual or oral intercourse.

Give Non-Sexual Affection

If you have to abstain from sex for an extended period of time, try to find other ways to maintain intimacy. Pay each other compliments, give gifts, refrain from criticism, or plan a fun date. Non-sexual affection can go a long way to communicate unconditional love to each other.

Pain

*The physically painful effects of sex (and the emotional and
spiritual issues that developed from this) made for such a hard
time truly understanding each other.*
—Annabelle

Usually, any pain you may experience when you first start having sex
will gradually fade away, especially if you stretch your vagina before
marriage, use sufficient lubrication, and make sure that you're turned
on before having sex. But if your pain persists more than a month or
two after your honeymoon night, there may be an underlying physical
or psychological issue that needs addressing.

Tell Your Husband about the Pain

Women often refrain from telling their husbands about their pain
because they know it will upset their husbands or because they don't
want their husbands to have to stop having sex. But as someone who
loves you, these are very natural feelings for him! How awful to think
that his own pleasure is causing you pain! Don't hide this from him, but
let him love you by quickly stopping the thing that is hurting you. There
are plenty of other ways you can still be intimate with each other!

See a Doctor

If sex is still painful after a couple months, it's important for you to see
a doctor right away. There may be physical causes for this pain, and a
doctor can find ways of treating them so that this pain subsides. If your
doctor maintains that pain during sex is normal for women, find
another doctor.

Find a Godly Counselor

Sometimes the underlying issue is psychological. Whether it's negative experiences in your past or pain associated with sex in your present relationship, this can be a huge roadblock to enjoying sex with your husband. Many women have found healing with the help of a godly counselor. Therapy is a wonderful tool!

Sin

We did too many things before we got married that we shouldn't have. So I just thought our sex life was always going to be horrible—that God wasn't going to bless our sex life since we messed up before marriage. But that's just not true.
—Violet

Sex is meant to mirror the intimacy that was once found in the garden of Eden when God would stroll side by side with Adam and Eve, delighting in their conversation, they marveling at his ideas, each full of love and openness toward the others. But much like the garden of Eden, that perfection no longer exists within sex.

Instead of open communication, we find the painful reality of angry outbursts and the silence of shame. Instead of complete vulnerability and availability, we feel the crushing weight of a rejected sexual advance. And even though we can intellectually acknowledge that sex is good and godly, we still hear a small voice whispering our guilt.

Our world is broken, bent, and lopsided—ravaged by the effects of sin. No one's sex life is perfect. No married couple—no matter how wise, passionate, or pure—experiences ideal sex. This is a rude awakening for many of us who unconsciously had looked to marriage to save us. We had hoped to find perfect satisfaction, comfort, and love in marriage, but because of sin, this is now impossible.

But it is here, at our lowest point, when we see the great power of God's redemptive work.

The Cross Breaks the Power of Sin

When Jesus died on the cross, suffering the punishment for our sin, he broke the power of sin over our lives. Because of Jesus's righteousness imparted to you, you need not fear the punishment for all the times you have sinned against your husband. You no longer look to your own goodness, to your marriage, or to sex to save you, because Jesus has saved you by his grace.

The Cross Gives You the Power to Show Grace

It does this in two different ways. First, once you comprehend the enormous debt that God has forgiven you, it becomes much easier to forgive whatever smaller debt your husband owes you. Secondly, when you understand that Jesus paid the debt that your husband owes you, there is no longer any reason to hold that grudge. Again, because Jesus suffered the punishment for your sins against each other, there is no longer anything standing in the way for complete reconciliation with each other.

The Cross Gives You the Power to Change

When you accept Jesus' atoning sacrifice for your sins, he promises to place the Holy Spirit in your heart to change your heart so that it desires to be like God. In Ezekiel 36:25–27 (ESV), God says, "I will sprinkle clean water on you, and you shall be clean from all your uncleannesses, and from all your idols I will cleanse you. And I will give you a new heart, and a new spirit I will put within you. And I will remove the heart of stone from your flesh and give you a heart of flesh. And I will put my Spirit within you, and cause you to walk in my statutes and be careful to obey my rules."

When it comes to the painful effects of sin, we need only look at the cross to see that God hasn't required us to figure out how to clean up our own mess. Even though it's our fault that our marriages are messed up and our sex lives littered with guilt and pain, God has cleaned it up for us. He's done all the work, and we need only to live our lives as though this were true . . . because it is! When we trust that God has made provision for our sin, when we choose not to punish those who sin against us, and we let God change our hearts so that we desire to be like him, then we most fully embrace our calling as darlings—a life lived as those loved by God.

Suggested Reading

I knew almost nothing before I got engaged. Zilch. Nada. Nothing. However, once I got engaged I went on a pretty serious quest to get informed. I talked to my doctor, my married friends, my older sister-in-law. I read books and magazines. I talked with my fiancé about it. Eventually, both my mom and my dad had a conversation with me that had good information. All these things helped me have an idea of what was going to happen and ways to help us in the beginning.

—Nancy

We had one of those God Made Sex and It's Awesome books. (We had to throw away one book that actually had pictures of people in positions. So we found one with drawings.) In the book were positions you might not think about . . . there were topics you should discuss . . . having a book and reading it together is kind of like having a premarital counselor. Once you're married and having sex, having read the book will help open up dialogue when it might otherwise be awkward.

—Miriam

There are so many helpful books and articles about sex. Read them. Even if you're not into reading, this is the best way to get informed. Please don't confuse ignorance with innocence. Spend time reading so that you're prepared for this grand new journey.

Here are a few great books from a godly perspective that contain loads of helpful information on sex, womanhood, and living as a darling of God:

- *Real Sex: The Naked Truth About Chastity* by Lauren F. Winner
- *A Celebration of Sex: A Guide to Enjoying God's Gift of Sexual Intimacy* by Dr. Douglas E. Rosenau or *A Celebration of Sex for Newlyweds* by Dr. Douglas E. Rosenau
- *The Act of Marriage: The Beauty of Sexual Love* by Tim and Beverly LaHaye
- *Sheet Music: Uncovering the Secrets of Sexual Intimacy in Marriage* by Kevin Leman
- *The Meaning of Marriage: Facing the Complexities of Commitment with the Wisdom of God* by Timothy and Kathy Keller
- *Sacred Marriage: What If God Designed Marriage to Make Us Holy More Than to Make Us Happy?* by Gary Thomas
- *You Can Change: God's Transforming Power for Our Sinful Behavior and Negative Emotions* by Tim Chester
- *Emotionally Healthy Spirituality: It's Impossible to Be Spiritually Mature, While Remaining Emotionally Immature* by Peter Scazzero

Honeymoon Stories

There are a million different ways your honeymoon night can play out, and you won't be able to predict what will happen. The following contains a number of honeymoon stories from Christian women. Read these with as little judgment as possible. Instead of seeing the stories as good or bad, try to view them as possibilities, understanding that you won't know how you or your husband will respond to the honeymoon night, because you haven't been there together yet!

Mia

After a record time of only an hour and ten minutes at our own reception, we peaced out! Since we were flying out of a different city, we decided to change clothes and leave our wedding attire behind before hitting the road.

Being the control freak I am, I didn't want the first time my husband saw me to be in my mother's house while I was a hot, stinky mess. I know. I regret not just going with it! On our way to Tulsa, we were a bit handsy. Longest forty minutes ever!

After checking in to our beautiful hotel, showers were in order. Again with the controlling, I wanted us to be clean and I did not want my husband to smell how I really smell after sweating for fifteen-plus hours on a hot summer day! He went first.

While he showered, I devoured both of our containers of food that were sent with us. Apparently, I wasn't too nervous, considering the way I ate! I showered and then donned my white pretty I had been gifted. I felt so giddy and so cheesy at the same time, but I had always imagined in my head how I wanted my husband to see me for the first time.

I remember so vividly the look of desire and love on my husband's face. It never felt awkward after that! I remember him undressing me and looking at me for the first time. I remember seeing and feeling him for the time. I remember commenting to him, "It's so soft!"

That night we just used our hands and the very tip of him. We were both able to orgasm that night. We then cuddled and fell asleep together! We had already decided during our counseling that we would take our time and not force it so it wouldn't be a painful experience. Each time we were able to go further and further. One and a half weeks later, my husband made it all the way in. It was a proud moment for us both!

Savannah

I was absolutely terrified of having sex. I had heard horror stories of pain, blood, and awkwardness, so our wedding night was not something I was looking forward to.

The DJ at our reception had to play the song "Kokomo" about six times before I would actually leave. Once we got in the car and Ian started driving toward the hotel, I panicked again and said the first thing I could think of to stall, "Can we please go to Sonic?! I need a vanilla Dr. Pepper!"

He kindly obliged (knowing full well how badly I was freaking out), so off to Sonic we went. Thankfully he wasn't too familiar with my hometown, so I was able to navigate us to one clear across town instead of one a few blocks away. I'm pretty sure he still doesn't know about that detail. We got our drinks and headed back to the hotel.

Once we went inside, we realized Ian's best man and his wife had left us a basket with a sweet note and a bottle of champagne. Ian went in and took a shower first while I drank some champagne and stood nervously staring (not sitting on, just staring) at the bed.

When he finished, I went in and took a shower and put on my wedding night lingerie. The shower and champagne did wonders for my nerves. I was so much calmer after that.

We got in bed and did a lot of kissing and cuddling. Thanks to the champagne, it's all a bit of a blur. We had sex, but I was so tight that it was difficult for him to enter. To be honest, it hurt pretty badly. I tried to hide the fact that it was painful because I was bound and determined to have sex on our wedding night, and I knew he would stop if he could tell I was uncomfortable. Thankfully, we made it through!

It hurt more than I anticipated, but it was more wonderful than I could have imagined. I loved our wedding night and was so thankful to know that I was going to wake up with my husband and that the pain and nervousness didn't even matter.

Sex was pretty painful for me the whole time we were on our honeymoon. I was scared to move or to do anything that would add pain, so I was pretty still every time. One day Ian stopped and said, "Babe, I love having sex with you. It's amazing. But could you please touch me with your arm, or move, or do anything at all? It feels like I'm doing a blow-up doll here."

We laughed for a good five minutes after that. It was awkward, but it's something we still laugh about today. I was so glad he actually said something instead of me just dealing with it because I wanted it to be a good experience for him.

I was prepared that sex wasn't going to be like it is in the movies. I knew it was going to be slightly awkward and things wouldn't go as smoothly as I had hoped. However, I think I may have been over prepared for it to be terrible. Instead of having any hope that it would be romantic and intimate, I was so focused on the negative that it took me a few weeks to start remembering that sex is a fun and enjoyable thing. I am forever grateful for the friends who gave me warnings, but I wish someone would have told me some positives as well.

Also, don't be afraid to get a little tipsy on your wedding night. A glass of champagne calmed me down so much, and I was very thankful for that. The more stressed you are, the more difficult it's going to be.

I enjoyed sleeping in the same bed. I appreciated that even more than sex. On our wedding night, Ian woke me up in the middle of the night just to say, "Hey, remember how we're sleeping together? I just don't want to forget how amazing this is." And it really was.

Gabriella

My husband was surprised that I wanted to leave our reception and "get to it" quicker than he did! We drove to a nearby town to a theme hotel, we were giddy the whole way, as it was hard to express that we were about to do it.

He took a shower, and I waited near the bed because he wanted to take off my wedding dress. I wish I hadn't had so many gazillion tiny buttons on it!

We kept the lights lowered/off. (He was the one who described to me what happens to a guy when he gets aroused . . . he was the first one to tell me . . . in a Target . . . when we were engaged.) He was so gentle as we touched each other in the dark first.

Because I was a virgin and hadn't done any stretching, it was painful, and it took four days for us to finish. Yep—we were in a different hotel, different place, before we could finish off. Poor guy, but it was one of the most profound things I remember, because he was so patient and gentle, tender and intimate, and we were creative.

One of the most vulnerable experiences was when my husband told me he wanted me shaved down there on our wedding night . . . and asked to do it. It was our first night married, and I knew we were doing something that was our own story. It was so new to me, both the concept of being shaved and having a man touch me. We laughed and it was so incredibly bonding. It was vulnerable, intimate, sexual, and almost as profound as the act itself. Who'd have thought?!

Bella

My husband and I planned to have the evening and night together, rather than showing up to our hotel super late and then driving and flying the next day without our sanity. On our forty-five-minute drive over I remember having no idea what would take place and yet knowing I should have a certain feeling because what was about to happen was going to be so monumental. I can't even tell you what we talked about besides the wedding, but I do know my husband was telling me how excited he was to see my body. Unfortunately, I was so not in the right mind-set that all I wanted to do was be with him and sleep in the same bed. I had this false picture of sex that I needed help repainting, and I didn't even know it.

I remember enjoying our dinner/snack and undressing. I cannot tell you exactly what happened next, but I think it was something like this. We, as most first-time lovers, I'm sure, were so starstruck by each other and everything was so new that each step had to be communicated. (Oh, the movies.)

I'm not even sure there was much fondling going on, and that was the problem. I didn't know how to be turned on, what that meant, and that I needed to relax. We just went right for sex. Because he went right in, of course I tore, and I knew right then and there something was wrong. I thought, "This thing was supposed to be so beautiful and right, but it feels so strange and not fun. God created this?"

I'm generally a pessimist, but that night my husband assured me that we would work it out. We were determined that if we just fixed a few things or kept doing it, sex would eventually turn out right.

That night my husband, like myself, was content to just stop and enjoy each other's company in the fun room (we had a rainforest-themed room), the hot tub, and we laughed at the hilarious rainforest animal noises that turn on and off with the switch.

The rest of the week was just painful as far as sex goes, but otherwise, I very much enjoyed my new life.

Willa

We did not have sex on our wedding night. We tried to, but it was really uncomfortable for me. We hadn't had sex before we got married, and we didn't use any lubrication (because I didn't know I would need it).

It was also really late, and we had had some champagne. I was just ready to go to sleep and really wasn't in the mood. I just wanted to crash!

So we just went to sleep, and I know Aaron was let down. I definitely recommend couples talk about their expectations for the wedding night and not to put a lot of pressure to have sex after the wedding. If you're both up for it, then go ahead, but I think it would be so much better to cuddle and talk about the night and then get a good night's sleep. Wake up and have sex! That's just what I would have wanted from my experience!

Charlotte

We went to a really nice hotel, and I remember I was on my period. I tried to prevent it using birth control, but it didn't work out. He was really cool about my period because he was just excited to have sex. He said, "It's not like I've ever done it before, so I won't know the difference."

We made out and tried to have sex, but I wasn't quite ready. He said, "Let's take a shower together." So we took a hot shower together, and then we were way more relaxed, and we had sex. And it was great. We were both on our sides, facing each other. I think that's funny, because now we never do it that way, but at the time it just seemed like the easiest way.

And then I remember we woke up at four in the morning and had sex again. We were just sleeping, and when our bodies touched each other it was like there was an electric shock. We were like, "Whee! We can have sex again!"

I feel like our honeymoon went really well. I didn't have pain or anything like that. I didn't stretch myself out beforehand, either. That may sound bad, like Sam's penis is tiny or something. But it was all just really enjoyable.

Stella

We checked in to our hotel and ordered some drinks at the bar, trying to decide what to do for dinner. We were on the opposite side of town from all the restaurants, so we opted for room service. Then we couldn't decide if we wanted to order dinner "before" or "after." We went ahead and ordered, and then started making out while we were waiting. We had both shed a few layers when the room service showed up, so there was a longer-than-normal awkward wait before we opened the door (awkward for me anyway!).

We got our food in the room, then got back down to business. We actually made it all the way, which I had been warned by a few of my girlfriends might not happen, so go, Mason! Then we ate our cold room service dinner in the hot tub.

I was a tiny bit sore after the very first time, but no problems. We never even needed lube.

Ellen

Well, we couldn't wait until we got to our hotel, which was forty-five minutes away from the location of our reception. We had a limousine that was driving us there, and we had already changed out of our wedding clothes.

So we rolled up the divider between us and the driver and had sex in the backseat. I don't know if the driver heard or saw anything—

probably not because it only lasted about two and a half minutes—but if he did, he played it cool and didn't mention it. It was very awkward, with lots of fumbling and slipping and falling all over the leather seat. When we got to our hotel room, there were champagne and strawberries waiting for us, along with a big whirlpool tub. We took a bath together, drank the champagne, and went another round. This one was slightly longer and much less awkward.

Emma

While we were engaged, we read Song of Solomon. We decided we would stop at a certain point (where it got juicy) and save that for our wedding night. So as soon as we got to our bridal suite, we read the rest of Song of Solomon. It was a sweet moment knowing that God created and cares about intimacy and that sex can be such a beautiful experience. I'm pretty sure we were both naked when we read it, which made it much more exciting! Then I know we took a shower together and just explored each other's bodies. It was quite interesting trying to have sex for the first time and making everything "fit," but we did it!

At one point, I modeled each of the new lingerie pieces I got, and he wasn't allowed to touch me at all—just look—and then he picked his favorite. And then I think for the last one I came out naked.

Julia

We had already talked about our expectations, desires, fears, and insecurities way before the wedding week so that we had time to process and plan.

We got married an hour away from where we stayed that first night so that we could fly out early the following morning for the remainder of our honeymoon. I will never forget when we arrived at our hotel, I was filled with excitement and nerves. We got up to our room, and we walked around to see everything. Since we had danced the night away at our reception, Adam decided he wanted to shower. Whew! Pressure was off! Praise the Lord.

While he showered, I got dressed and situated, which made the rest of the night so comfortable. I knew that I was going to have to break the ice, so as soon as I heard the shower stop, I jumped in the closet to surprise Adam. I heard him walk around our suite (which was so funny). He finally got close enough to the closet that I popped it open, stood in a sexy pose with my sexy outfit on, and said, "Wanna make out and see where it leads?"

Of course that broke the ice, made us both laugh, and got things moving quickly. We took things slow and communicated how the other was feeling the whole time. We had the lights semi-off so we could see each other, but it wasn't bright. We called it our mood lighting, which we still prefer.

Did it last forever? Of course not. Ha! My husband was a twenty-six-year-old virgin, but it was perfect. We spent the rest of the night making out, cuddling, and talking. We didn't have sex all night but spent the night recapping all of our favorite parts of our wedding and what we looked forward to doing together the rest of our honeymoon in Mexico.

My honeymoon night wasn't painful at all. It actually was more painful later that week because we had been having sex so much that my vagina felt like it had been beat up! But it subsided soon after.

Fiona

We had an early wedding, then stopped and got some snacks and a bottle of champagne before heading to our bed-and-breakfast. We got there around 7:00 p.m., nice and early, so we weren't exhausted already.

We had already talked beforehand about what we wanted the night to look like (for example, music/not music, lighting, smells, tastes, expectations from both sides, etc.). So we went into it quite prepared.

(However, we turned our music off about halfway through deciding neither of us were a big fan.)

So I went and got dressed (in special lingerie) and ready in the bathroom. He went and got ready on the bed. I wanted his eyes to be closed when I came out. So I came around behind him on the bed and touched his back a bit. He turned around and it all began. We just looked at each other, studied each other, touched each other, went very slowly, put a pillow under my lower back (as was told by many sources), and went from there . . .

It all went smoothly.

Gemma

We got away from the reception as quickly as possible. We flew to Chicago for our honeymoon and didn't arrive until 10:00 p.m. We were exhausted. (On the plane, we asked for a blanket and fondled each other the whole way there.)

When we first arrived at our honeymoon place, because we were so tired, Landon started giggling about everything. I was trying to be all sexy, and he was giggling. It was soooo not the right response when I was getting naked.

Just then, the hotel sent up champagne, but when they knocked on the door, we were both in stages of undress. I sprinted to the bathroom while he pulled on his pants. The champagne helped us relax, though.

Grace

We were wired when we got in our car to drive away from the wedding. Our hotel was sixty miles away. I think we arrived in less than forty-five minutes. Even on the drive, we started touching each other, hardly able to wait.

Soon, we made it to our room. I had purposely kept my wedding dress on because I wanted him to take it off of me. When he took off my dress he stepped back and said, "You're like a super model." That was maybe the most perfect thing he could've said in that moment.

By the time I got his pants off, his penis was so big. I realized, all of a sudden, that I'd never seen an erect penis. I kept thinking, "Is this what they actually look like?" Then I began to have serious doubts as to whether or not it could fit inside me. But I remember trying really hard not to look shocked or scared. Maybe I should've expressed my awe at how big he was and given him a similarly perfect moment.

We started kissing slowly and passionately, but when he came into me we stopped kissing and started talking. He went slowly, kept asking me how it felt and I told him. It hurt. But it wasn't unbearable, and I urged him to keep pushing. I just told him to go really, really slowly.

Here I encountered an unexpected problem. The pain almost immediately made all my pleasure sensors turn off. It was like I was turned on and turned off, all at the same time.

I was confused, and he felt unhappy that it didn't feel good for me. After a few moments the pain wasn't as severe and I could start feeling him inside me. This helped to increase the pleasure of it, but I was never able to relax enough to have an orgasm. He did, which made me so happy, but he was disconcerted that I didn't.

Afterward we cuddled and kissed and did a recap. Then we both just got right in the shower together. The heat and steam helped me to relax. It all felt so sexy under the water, and we began to kiss again. And we had sex again.

And once again, it hurt. But it hurt less, and I was able to feel a little bit more pleasure.

Sometime later that night, I got out my pretty box of lingerie. I came out of the bathroom all pretty, and when we had sex this time, I orgasmed.

Acknowledgments

From beginning to end, this book was surrounded by the encouragement, support, help, advice, expertise, and generosity of many people.

I can't fully express my gratitude to the women who allowed me to interview them about their sex lives. Their bravery, transparency, and humble willingness to share their stories in the hopes that it might help other women was an inspiration to me. Their names have been changed to protect their privacy, but their effect on this book cannot be overstated.

Many thanks to Dr. Cheryl Fogarty, OB/GYN, Dr. Peter Buckland, and Melissa Winston for giving me the time of day and allowing me to pick their brains. Their expertise and wisdom were invaluable.

Many friends read the book and helped in the editing process. I'd especially like to thank Ellie Lang, Rebeca Berry, and Chris Wheeler for so generously giving their time to go over this book with a fine-toothed comb. It's so much better because of them!

Thanks to Sarah Hester for her brilliant design work and all those encouraging emojis. Her cheerleading has been such a bright spot in this journey.

Deb Hall was the best editor a woman could ask for. She understood my vision for this project, worked her magic, and handed it back all tidy, clean, and glittering.

I'd like to thank Logan, my dear husband and friend. Not only was this book his idea in the first place, but he was there every step of the way with encouraging words, good ideas, a helping hand, and countless hours of designing and brainstorming. He is my inspiration, in every possible way.

Finally, I'd like to thank the amazing women in my life. Many thanks to my mom, for her love and teaching through the years, and for her example of a woman who wasn't ashamed of a good kiss. Thanks to my sisters for talking with me about everything. I learned to enjoy the company of good women from them and am still learning from each of them. Finally, I want to thank my Girls' Night girls. Meeting once a month, eating delicious food, and talking about every subject under the sun has been one of the more meaningful experiences of my life. It made me realize that instead of being the source of comparison, insecurity, and jealousy, as is so often the case, talking with other women about sex can be helpful, inspiring, and comforting. They are the best of women.

About the Author

Aanna Greer is a writer, speaker, wife, and mother whose passion is connecting women to God and to each other. With over ten years of youth and college ministry, and experience teaching sex ed in the public school system, she loves to help women understand and embrace their sexuality. Aanna lives in southwest Missouri with her husband and two daughters, where she can usually be found with a coffee in one hand and a book in the other.

Notes

Introduction

1. C. John Collins, "Psalms" in *The ESV Study Bible*, eds. Lane T. Dennis et al. (Wheaton: Crossway, 2008), 945.
2. "Darling," Merriam-Webster.com, accessed February 9, 2017, https://www.merriam-webster.com/dictionary/darling.

Chapter 1: God's Design for Sex

3. F. Scott Fitzgerald, *The Great Gatsby* (New York: Scribner, 2004), 180.
4. Timothy and Kathy Keller, *The Meaning of Marriage: Facing the Complexities of Commitment with the Wisdom of God* (New York: Dutton, 2011), 224.
5. See Lauren F. Winner, *Real Sex: The Naked Truth about Chastity* (Grand Rapids: Brazos Press, 2005), 37–38.
6. Phil Spector, "To Know Him Is to Love Him," single recorded by the Teddy Bears, Doré Records, 1958.
7. Denny Burk, *What Is The Meaning of Sex?* (Wheaton: Crossway, 2013), 38.

Chapter 3: Caring for Your Body

8. Melissa Conrad Stöppler, MD, "Yeast Infection (in Women and Men)," accessed April 7, 2017, http://www.medicinenet.com/yeast_infection_in_women_and_men/article.htm which cites an article by Linda O. Eckert, "Acute vulvovaginitis," New England Journal of Medicine 355 (2006): 1244-1252.

Chapter 4: How to Be a Darling When You're Single

9. This perspective on boundaries relies heavily on Lauren F. Winner's story in "On the Steps of the Rotunda," from *Real Sex: The Naked Truth about Chastity* (Grand Rapids: Brazos Press, 2005), 107–108.

10. Michael Reece, Debby Herbenick, J. Dennis Fortenberry, Brian Dodge, Stephanie A. Sanders, Vanessa Schick, "National Survey of Sexual Health and Behavior," accessed January 5, 2017, http://www.nationalsexstudy.indiana.edu/graph.html.

11. Douglas E. Rosenau, *A Celebration of Sex: A Guide to Enjoying God's Gift of Sexual Intimacy* (Nashville: Thomas Nelson, 2002), 309.

12. "Shame," Merriam-Webster.com, accessed February 15, 2017, https://www.merriam-webster.com/dictionary/shame.

13. The ideas in this section on Christ's desire to remove shame relies heavily on a roundtable discussion with Trillia Newbell, Scotty Smith, and Justin Holcomb titled "Caring for Victims of Sexual Abuse," accessed January 5, 2017, http://resources.thegospelcoalition.org/library/caring-for-victims-of-sexual-abuse.

14. Cameron Cole, "Rethinking Sex Ed in the Church," www.thegospelcoalition.com, accessed June 5, 2015, https://www.thegospelcoalition.org/article/rethinking-sex-ed-in-the-church.

Chapter 5: How to Be a Darling When You're Engaged

15. 2014 Proven Men Porn Survey (conducted by Barna Group), Proven Men Ministries, accessed April 12, 2017, www.provenmen.org/2014pornsurvey.

16. *Pornographic* (Joplin: Choices Medical Services, 2014).

17. *You, Me & Porn* (Joplin: Choices Medical Services, 2014).

18. "Condoms and Pregnancy Prevention," SexEdLibrary.Org, Sexuality Education Council of the United States, accessed September 15, 2017, http://www.sexedlibrary.org/index.cfm?pageId=788

Chapter 7: The Basics of Sex

19. Lauren F. Winner, *Real Sex: The Naked Truth about Chastity* (Grand Rapids: Brazos Press, 2005), 42.